Everything CBD:

How to Buy - Use - Grow - Invest
in
Cannabis

R.J. Stewart

Table of Contents

—

Introduction

Global public perception about the benefits of using cannabis is dramatically changing with more international jurisdictions moving to legalize recreational marijuana and decriminalize its possession.

As we begin to understand more about what this incredible plant can do, more people are exploring how cannabis can help them with their specific health challenges. Like beer and wine, this is proof that God loves us and wants us to be happy.

Just the other day I heard a story about a chicken and an egg. The chicken and the egg were lying in bed one afternoon. The chicken had its head on the pillow looking very content while smoking a marijuana joint. The egg rolled over appearing very annoyed and said, "Well, I guess we answered that question?"

Unlike the chicken and the egg, you probably have a myriad of questions about cannabis that you would like answered. Like the chicken, they should come easy. This resource will answer many of your queries about how to buy, use, grow and invest in cannabis.

You'll find that this guide provides you with easy-to-follow, step-by-step approaches to four of the most common topics as it relates to cannabis. More specifically you'll enter the world of cannabidiol (CBD) one of the many therapeutically beneficial cannabinoids found in marijuana.

This resource is founded on current best practices, along with the latest developments and research into CBD use and production. We're seeing rapid change in this growing industry with new insights into what it can and cannot do. Technological advances into the production and processing of cannabis are allowing a plethora of CBD-rich products to enter the global market.

But with so much information out in the markets, how do you wade through all the hype surrounding the industry to make the right educated decisions? While wracking my hamster brain, I decided to share as much "actionable" research-based information with you as possible. You'll quickly discover that this resource focuses on "how to" get things done.

All of the material presented in this book has been tried and tested. You'll pick up sage advice from an assortment of industry leaders. In an attempt to minimize generalities, specific recommendations are given. And where possible extensive product and informational links are included to help you make better informed decisions that might affect your life.

As you read through your guide, you'll discover why I've selected CBD as the focal point of this book, as opposed to the more common cannabinoid THC.

So, what in God's pajamas can you expect to learn from this particular book? The book is divided into four major sections. Each section is organized so that you can use it as a stand-alone resource.

The first section explores what's so special about cannabis and specifically CBD. You'll find out what the U.S. and Canadian government's position is on marijuana. And you'll learn about those who can use cannabis safely and those who should avoid it.

The second section takes a look at how to legally buy cannabis products and from which general categories of cannabis products you'll be able to choose. I'll be sharing with you what CBD-rich cannabis varieties are the best to buy and for which common ailments they can have a positive effect. You'll also learn how to use the various products described in this section along with some specific dosing guidelines.

The third section shows you how to set up an inexpensive, discrete, closet grow and what it would take to grow successful crop after successful crop. You'll even learn how to make your own products, which could save you a pretty penny down the road. Or an ugly one for that matter.

Finally, section four taps into the world of investing and how you could become a part of this growing industry. Whether you're looking for a potential career change or starting up a cannabis-related business, money-making opportunities abound. I'll show you how to invest in individual stocks and create a monthly income stream by "renting" out your stock. With Canada poised to be a dominant player in world production and major US companies looking at tapping into this growing market, there's no better time than now to invest.

If you're curious about what CBD can do for you or you're a current cannabis user with unanswered questions that has a desire to do more for yourself, then this resource is for you.

And how do you make the most of your read? If you're new to CBD, I would suggest reading the material in sequential order. The topics are organized in such a manner that you may only wish to read the first two sections. This would allow you time to act on the recommendations and wait until you're ready to explore the sections on growing or investing.

Should you already have a good knowledge base, then skimming through the first two sections or jumping to a section that interests you may make more sense.

Whether you read through the book as outlined in sequential order or explore specific topics of interest, please take some time to explore the website links provided. None of the links are associated with any "affiliate marketing" programs. As well, re-read any chapters for clarity or email me if you get into a pickle.

Ready to see what's so special about cannabis?

Section 1: What's So Special about Cannabis?

This short introductory section, answers the following questions:
1. What's the relationship between cannabinoids and terpenes?
2. What are Indica, Sativa and Ruderalis plants?
3. What are the U.S. and Canadian government's take on marijuana?
4. What are cannabinoids and why are they so important to the endo-cannabinoid system in your body?
5. What's all the fuss over CBD?
6. Is cannabis safe?

This section sets the tone for other sections that follow. We're often provided with information that is informative yet lacks one key component - Is what is being discussed going to provide me with actionable tips? The focus of this particular book does just that. It takes you by the hand and explains how to buy, use, grow and invest in cannabis.

Let's jump right into addressing some common questions regarding cannabis.

Chapter 1: What is CBD?

Cannabis is one of the world's oldest cultivated plants for both its medicinal qualities and use for its fibers. It's an annual herb that is relatively tall and erect growing to a maximum height of 20 feet within a 4 to 6-month outdoor growing season. A more typical height for varieties grown in greenhouses or indoor facilities for medicinal purposes is under 5 feet.

Cannabis likes air that is warm, humid and rich in carbon dioxide. It grows well when water is abundant, yet not excessive and there is a constant supply of nutrients. Unlike grapes which thrive in nutritionally poor and arid soil conditions, cannabis prefers a more sub-tropical climate.

The plants are "dioecious" plants, meaning that they require both male and female flowers to propagate under normal environmental conditions. When planted in the spring, cannabis responds to increasing daylight with more vigorous vegetative growth. As fall approaches, shorter daylight hours trigger flowering to complete its life cycle. In the wild, wind pollinates the female plants. When this occurs, seeds are produced, fall to the ground and continue the life cycle. However, as budding consumers of marijuana, we want unpollinated, female plants to develop resinous glands containing cannabinoids, not seeds.

Cannabinoids and Terpenes:

The reason why cannabis has gained international attention is that it contains more than 200 different cannabinoids, of which 60 have promising medicinal and therapeutic capabilities. These cannabinoids are concentrated in glandular trichomes, which appear on floral clusters and those leaves located close to the clusters or buds.

They also contain 30 terpenes of note, which combine with cannabinoids in ways that affect how they're being absorbed and used by the body. This is precisely why the man-made, THC-based pharmaceutical "Dronabinol" shows so many negative side effects and doesn't work as well as cannabis in its natural form. No synthetic drug can replace what Mother Nature has so generously created to heal and rejuvenate the body.

Incidentally, terpenes are aromatic chemical compounds found in all plants, such as flowers, fruits and vegetables. They are quite volatile and fragrant, giving marijuana it's strong odors of pine, citrus, diesel, sour, etc. Terpenes play an important role in interacting with cannabinoids to produce subtle variations in the medicinal effects of each plant. As future research continues in this area, we're bound to gain a greater understanding as to how all of these chemical compounds interact in the human body.

The two most talked-about cannabinoids are THC (tetrahydrocannabinol) and CBD (cannabidiol). THC is known for its ability to quickly act on the brain producing a psychoactive response. Varieties rich in THC tend to be mood-stimulating. You often hear about it being recommended for daytime use. CBD typically produces a calming effect on the entire body, as opposed to the typical "head high" with THC varieties containing high THC concentrations. Varieties high in CBD tend to be more sedative and relaxing and are often recommended for nighttime use.

Cannabinoids are present in all parts of the cannabis plant. The highest concentrations can be found in the mature buds, with lower concentrations in the seeds, leaves and roots. Ripe, resin-coated female flowers or buds is what is most highly prized from any medical grow.

If you've ever walked into a cannabis shop and been blown away by the choices of cannabis available, you're not alone. Hundreds of varieties are available. You may have been at odds trying to select a variety that delivers the right combination of cannabinoids to best meet your needs.

What's also confusing is the language around cannabis. How do we classify all of these varieties so that they make sense? We often here the use of the term Sativa to describe THC dominant varieties and Indica for CBD strains. Today we understand a heck of a lot more about this plant than 10 years ago. Much of the descriptors and labels used in the past have been debunked as myths. However, despite the latest genetic research in the field, the cannabis industry still uses these terms incorrectly. Which brings us to the ongoing debate between the terms, Sativa, Indica and Ruderalis.

Indica and Sativa plants:

Recent research in the past decade has pointed out that all cannabinoid-rich cannabis varieties share a narrow range of genes. And all of the hemp-fiber producing varieties another set of genes. Geneticists have recently classified the drug-producing varieties as Cannabis Indica, with the fiber varieties as being Cannabis Sativa. Yikes! That flies in the face of conventional terminology.

—

6

Indica plants have their origins along the 30th parallel of the India sub-continent in countries stretching across Afghanistan, Pakistan, Tajikistan and northern India. This climatic zone tends to be more variable in its weather patterns year to year. Since plants had to adjust to fluctuating temperature, humidity and light levels, they adapted by showing a high degree of heterogeneity resulting in lots of variability within that variety's population. This helps the population survive, despite the changing weather patterns.

Now within the Indica varieties, you have both broad and narrow-leafed plants. Many cannabinoid-rich varieties in the marketplace today are a hybrid of the two sub-classifications, with most varieties having a broad-leafed appearance. Broad-leafed plants arose to capture more of the sun's rays, especially in growing regions well above the equator. The plants tend to have dark-green, colored leaves that enable them to capture sunlight more efficiently under lower light conditions. They're also shorter, bushier and more compact.

Medicinal sativa plants arose in countries situated between the equator and the 20th parallel, like Thailand, Jamaica, Nigeria and Columbia. These plants were initially brought to these regions to produce hemp fiber that could be used in the textile and building industries. The original fiber-producing, root stock came from sativa plants grown in temperate regions around the world between the 40th and 50th parallels. Over the course of several hundred years of selective breeding, sativa plants have been grown more for their medicinal qualities. As word-wide hemp use and production declined, growers started replacing industrial hemp with a cash crop having sought-after medicinal properties.

Fiber-producing sativa plants (the original hemp plants) typically produce more CBD and less than 1% THC. You may have come across topical CBD oils, creams and lotions produced from processing huge quantities of hemp. These medicinal products are often labeled as Hemp Oil.

What's really important about these insights and on-going debate is not the specific classification of what you're buying and using, it's the chemical breakdown of the cannabinoid levels that truly matters to you at the end of the day. What you're more interested in is whether or not a particular cannabis product will help you. Am I correct?

Ruderalis plants:

The term Ruderalis gained notoriety back in the late 1920's. It is a variant of cannabis alongside Sativa and Indica. Botanists disagree as to whether or not Ruderalis qualifies as a species, sub-species or variant. These plants were discovered growing wild in areas north of the 40th parallel in western Asia. They had the distinct ability to automatically flower. Most cannabis plants require a change in the light cycle for the plants to begin flowering. As the days grow shorter and cooler, the plants look to self-preservation through reproduction. The production of flowers in the female plant and pollen by the male plant ensures that the life cycle of the species continues.

What's important to know about the Ruderalis plant is that it's being genetically crossed by breeders with Indica plants to create auto-flowering varieties. Being shorter in size, it matures much faster than most Indicas or Sativas. This characteristic is also being passed on to the new hybrids being created. In the ever-changing world of medical marijuana production, new hybrids are being created that grow faster to maturity in smaller spaces and produce higher concentrations of cannabinols, making indoor production that much more feasible.

What's the origin of cannabis?

The first documented cases of the use of cannabis in society date back over 5000 years. It has appeared in the records of the Egyptians, Greeks, Indians, and Chinese. Of interest, is a burial tomb of a local shaman in China dating back to 2700 BC that contained nearly two pounds of cannabis. Imagine the send-off he had at his wake.

All through the 1840's and up to the 1920's, cannabis was being widely prescribed to help with pain, upper respiratory ailments and depression. It wasn't until this last century where we've experienced an all-out war on the plant globally.

—

What's the Government's take on marijuana?

In the 1930's, the US government began regulating cannabis, coincidently at the same time as the alcohol prohibition era. Marijuana was outright banned in 1937 with the Marijuana Tax Act. And in 1970 it was classified as a "Schedule 1" drug, meaning that it was deemed to have no medicinal benefits. This meant that it could no longer be grown and studied, unless Federal approval was granted. Cannabis went from being touted as having healing qualities and being a safe and effective medicine to being banned as a dangerous narcotic without the scientific evidence to support the claim. Are you as confused as a dog who just saw a card trick? Go figure!

In 1964, the tipping point for the modern era of cannabis research occurred in Israel when tetrahydrocannabinol (THC) was isolated. Since then dozens of beneficial and promising compounds have been identified in the plant. And with greater wisdom about the plant comes greater acceptance globally.

Despite opposition at the federal level, a growing number of states have legalized medical marijuana. West Virginia became the 29th state to do so in 2017. On October 17, 2018 Canada legalized the recreational use of marijuana, making it one of a handful of nations recognizing the positive benefits of cannabis on a national scale. Mexico is slated to follow suit in decriminalizing marijuana and recognizing the medicinal benefits of this life-giving plant.

What's so alarming is the US Federal Government's refusal to acknowledge the health benefits of medicinal marijuana. The Federal Government continues to threaten US citizens who use cannabis with criminal charges. Isn't any Government supposed to work towards supporting the collective good of the nation and not suppress life-saving research or deny individuals access to medicine shown to improve the quality of life? I'm as confused as a homeless man under house arrest on this one.

Now should you be Canadian eh, the federal government has sent a clear message to the rest of the world that the legalization and decriminalization of cannabis is the future. Recreational use of cannabis is legal across Canada with adults being able to grow up to 4 plants per household for personal consumption and possess up to 100 grams of home-grown marijuana. Not only that, but extensive research can finally be conducted as to how we can receive the optimal benefits from this incredible plant. Both US and Canadian research companies have set up shop in Canada to do just that. This means that in just a few years' time Canada will be at the forefront of doing cutting edge research into the benefits of this wonderful plant. Imagine the investment opportunities that'll abound as a result.

What makes cannabis so special?

It's all in the resin. When an unpollinated female plant or "sinsemilla" seedless plant develops, the bulbous trichomes located on the flowers produce the highly, sought-after resin. This resin contains all that steamy goodness we want to help cure what ails us.

Trichomes evolved as a means for the plant to defend itself from pests and to help with the dispersal of pollen. The bulbous trichomes situated at the top of the plant in the flower clusters secrete cannabinoids, terpenes and fats as a sticky resin. Being delicate, they can easily rupture releasing terpenes that give the plant its distinctive odor. Once ruptured the cannabinoids are quickly oxidized losing their medicinal value. When the buds are harvested at their peak ripeness, carefully manicured and allowed to dry they contain the highest concentrations of medicine.

Cannabinoids and the Endo-Cannabinoid System:

The discovery of the endocannabinoid system that is found in all complex animals is a recent one, dating back to the late 80's. The system helps regulate the immune system, inflammation, pain, motor function, digestion, appetite, and memory. Like most biological systems, the endocannabinoid system (ECS) is comprised of three structural parts:
1. Endocannabinoid receptors.
2. Endocannabinoids.
3. Enzymes.

There are two primary types of endocannabinoid receptors, namely CB_1 and CB_2. Recent research has shown that both can be found throughout the body in various systems, like the:

1. nervous system,
2. immune system,
3. gastrointestinal system,
4. endocrine system,
5. circulatory system,
6. reproductive system, and the
7. brain.

Being present in so many systems makes you wonder about how important cannabinoids are in the day-to-day regulatory functions of the human body. Unfortunately, scientific research in the United States has been limited in this area. Most of the current scientific literature and discoveries are coming from countries that have a more liberal view about the positive role cannabis can serve in society. As we begin to understand more about the ECS, we'll be in a better position to process and prescribe cannabis products that'll specifically target certain health conditions.

There are currently two endocannabinoid receptors of note, CB_1 and CB_2. They are widely distributed throughout the body. Both CBD and THC bind with these two receptor sites to produce the physiological effects of cannabis. THC actively binds with CB_1 to produce a psychoactive response. Some researchers have suggested changing its name from CB_1 to THC receptor.

What's interesting to note, is that the body naturally produces chemical compounds called "anandamides" that activate cannabinoid receptors, not unlike what CBD and THC do. Research into anandamides, may give credibility to the age-old saying "getting high on life". The human body naturally takes advantage of its own internal chemistry for producing feel-good chemicals. The endocannabinoid system may very well be one such component.

What are Endocannabinoids?

Endocannabinoids are derivatives of polyunsaturated fatty acids, not unlike omega-3 fatty acids found in fish oil. And your mom has probably touted the benefits of taking fish oil supplements, right? Being fat-based they aren't soluble in water. The human body - as described by an alien - could be looked at as being "an ugly sack of mostly water". This means that endocannabinoids are not easily transported within the body. Because of this, the body tends to manufacture specific endocannabinoids that target select, local areas of the body.

When cannabinoids like THC and CBD from cannabis are either smoked or vaped, they bind with protein molecules in the blood plasma within minutes. They're distributed to regions of the body that have lots of blood vessels such as the heart, lungs and liver. Each of these tissues uses enzymes to slowly breaks down the cannabinoids, requiring about 48 hours to eliminate them from the bloodstream.

In their natural states, both THC and CBD exist in the form of acids. THCA and CBDA are converted into the active forms of THC and CBD with the application of heat. Smoking or vaping dried bud does this instantly. Cannabis that has been processed as a tincture, oil, or edible has undergone a heat conversion process called decarboxylation. Gentle heating of CBD-rich cannabis at 245°F and a slightly cooler temperature of 220°F for THCA, decarboxylates (removes the acidic component) within 40 minutes. Now the final product is in the active form (bioavailable), ready to be taken up by the body as a digestible.

There is some controversy over which forms of THC/ THCA and CBD/ CBDA are more bioavailable for the body to use from a medicinal point of view. More extensive research will be required to put this ongoing debate to rest.

Why such a fuss over CBD?

We've heard all about the psychoactive effect that THC can produce in the body. The infamous, euphoric "head high" has been talked about and sought after for decades. Growing weed to be smoked for recreational purposes was much of the focus in the 20th century.

Recently, in the 21st century we've seen a shift in interest to the myriad of medicinal benefits that CBD and other lesser-known cannabinoids possess. We've all heard the story about 5-year old Charlotte Figi, whose severe form of epilepsy became manageable with CBD. Individuals like actor Morgan Freeman, singer Olivia Newton-John, actor Patrick Stewart, and singer Melissa Etheridge have all publicly proclaimed the benefits of cannabis. Each of these individuals suffers from ailments that cannabis has helped.

As our understanding of how CBD interacts with the body in addressing pain, seizures, tremors, hunger, and mood grows, so does the movement towards producing more CBD-rich cannabis varieties. More cultivars are now looking at growing more CBD-rich crops to meet the growing demand for CBD-related products.

Until recently, CBD was primarily sold as hemp oil. Hemp contains virtually no THC (less than 0.3%) and small amounts of CBD (usually less than 4%). Grown on an industrial scale, enough "Hemp" oil can be extracted from the plants and is used primarily for topical applications.

A better source of CBD comes from Cannabis Indica plants that are grown for their higher concentrations of CBD, with some varieties producing concentrations as high as 20%. This is a more cost-effective way of obtaining the sought-after, medicinal components. In this case, the higher concentrations of "CBD" oil can be used both internally as an edible product and externally as a topical cream or ointment.

We're discovering that those CBD-rich varieties that also contain appreciable levels of THC are able to mitigate pain better than either cannabinoid on its own. This is one reason why, you may be best served by products produced from Cannabis Indica varieties, as opposed to Cannabis Sativa (hemp). Although, much of the focus of this book is on the health benefits primarily offered by CBD, I'll also point out where CBD/THC varieties may be helpful.

The big question: Is cannabis safe?

There have been no reported deaths attributed specifically to a cannabis overdose. The worst-case scenario for most users who over-indulge is that they'll pass out and possibly wake up in panic mode with a headache, dry mouth and being hungrier than a bear coming out of hibernation.

As with any medication, consultation with an experienced medical professional should be one's first course of action before indulging. The challenge is finding a healthcare professional who has the training and experience with cannabis. Unfortunately, most medical professionals lack the formal training to be able to offer up-to-date advice. The majority of universities do not currently provide their med students with an appropriate grounding in the medicinal benefits of cannabis.

Of greatest concern are potential interactions with other prescription drugs you may be taking. For example, CBD can inhibit enzyme activity of cytochrome P450 in the liver, which the body uses to metabolize certain prescription medications. Consulting your local pharmacist may help guide you in avoiding any adverse effects and getting the most out of your prescription meds. Be aware that cannabis products containing THC increase the effects of alcohol, benzodiazepines (ex. Valium), and opiates (ex. codeine). Avoid mixing the two.

The elderly or those new to cannabis may also express a concern when using THC-rich products for the first time. The psychoactive effect may be alarming or uncomfortable. In general, you'll see a higher number of negative side effects with THC than CBD, which is a "non-intoxicating" cannabinoid.

The most common negative side effects of using cannabis are dry mouth, itchy eyes, feelings of paranoia, being anxious, headaches and light-headedness. Depending on the variety you're using you may experience some of these less-desirable effects.

High concentrations of CBD can also create "couch lock", where your body relaxes completely as you melt into the couch. Not an ideal scenario if you're scheduled to run a marathon when this happens. However, it could be a great way to spend an evening watching re-runs from the 90's on TV. Wouldn't you agree?

Should you experience short-term psychological effects such as confusion, anxiety or panic often associated with THC-rich products, reduce your dosage and look for products that also contain CBD. CBD/THC blends may reduce some of these side effects. Of course, if these psychological symptoms escalate, seek medical attention right away.

Unlike opioid overdoses, cannabis does not cause respiratory depression resulting in death. In fact, those who use cannabis to manage pain often reduce or eliminate their need to use prescription pain killers.

Cannabis is a non-toxic substance that the body tolerates well even at high doses. However, this should not be misconstrued as being - more is better. In fact, "less" may lead to an increased effect. High doses of cannabinoids cause an imbalance in the endocannabinoid system. The body reacts by reducing endocannabinoid receptor density in the body. As a general rule of thumb for cannabis dosage, look to establishing a "minimum effective dose" to address the medicinal need. Also, establish the shortest possible course of treatment so as to reduce developing dose-tolerance issues. More on this in Section 2.

Should you accidentally overdose on a THC-rich product, you'll want to rest in a comfortable setting and drink plenty of fluids until the negative effects subside. Having someone with you while you may be experiencing hallucinations, paranoia, panic, rapid heartbeat or nausea can be comforting and reassuring. Fortunately, CBD-rich products are not psychoactive and don't create an overdose effect.

Is Cannabis safe for minors?

THC-rich cannabis should not be consumed by minors. An adolescent's developing brain is adversely affected by introducing any intoxicating chemical into the body, whether that be alcohol, opioids or THC. Long-term use of THC-rich cannabis amongst adolescents has shown to decrease memory and problem-solving abilities with an associated drop in IQ. The earlier you start, the worse your cognitive growth becomes.

What is reassuring is that cannabis has a low addiction rate of only around 9%. Incidentally, alcohol has an addiction rate that's 40% higher at 14% with heroin coming in at a whopping 23%. As with these and other addictive substances, the later you start, the less likely your risk of dependency later in life.

Bottom line? Minors should avoid these drugs or risk permanent brain damage.

What about my pregnancy?

If you're pregnant or breast-feeding, avoid cannabis altogether. Just as an adolescent's developing brain is negatively impacted by cannabis, so is your baby's developing body. Consider diet or other lifestyle treatments before resorting to cannabis to deal with nausea, depression or anxiety that's often associated with pregnancies. Your unborn or developing child's long-term health is more important than the short-term benefits you may receive.

What about my pets?

The market for pet therapeutics is growing, especially those products rich in CBD. More than 66% of dog owners and 64% of cat owners surveyed in 2016 felt that their pets benefited.

Recall that all complex animals - including humans and your furry friends - have an endocannabinoid system capable of producing and processing cannabinoids. It's built into your and your pet's body.

Unfortunately, there is a research void on what works, might work better or doesn't work when it comes to cannabis and pets. What we do know is that anecdotal evidence shows that CBD is safe for pets. On the other hand, the rise in THC toxicity and overdoses in pets ingesting THC-rich edibles is a concern.

Should you be considering using CBD to help improve the quality of life of your pet, do so after you've discussed an appropriate course of action with your vet. Often the vet will recommend a multi-modal approach to tackling your pet's health challenges.

Now that we've addressed some of the common concerns about cannabis use. let's explore how to buy and use cannabis to suit your needs in the following section. Alright?

Section 2: Buying and Using CBD.

In this section of your book, you'll explore a number of topics related to how to buy and use CBD-rich cannabis, namely:
1. How do I obtain a medical marijuana licence?
2. What types of cannabis products are available in the market?
3. How do I select quality dried cannabis?
4. What CBD-rich cannabis varieties may be the best to buy?
5. For which common ailments can CBD-rich cannabis have a positive effect?
6. How do I select a medical marijuana dispensary?
7. Should I purchase marijuana online?
8. Is Holistic Health Care the answer?
9. How do I use the different cannabis products out in the market?

Let's dive right into how to legally access cannabis products as a medical patient.

Chapter 2: How Do I Buy Cannabis Products (legally)?

Each legal jurisdiction across North America has their own set of rules and regulations you must abide by in order to legally purchase CBD-rich products or medical grade marijuana. The challenge is knowing what you can and should not do if you want to access cannabis through the legal channels provided in your local area.

In 2018, nine states and D.C allowed the sale of both medical and recreational marijuana. Canada also falls into the same boat on a national scale with each province having control over how the general public will access cannabis-related products. Access is much easier in these jurisdictions since you do not require a physician-prescribed medical marijuana licence. According to a CBS News poll in 2017, 61% of Americans felt that marijuana should be legal in general.

Currently an additional 20 states have approved the sale of medical marijuana to those individuals who have a medical marijuana card. An additional 15 states offer very limited access to CBD. Support for access to medical marijuana is growing steadily with 85% of Americans being in favor of legalizing marijuana for medical conditions. About time, wouldn't you agree?

How do I go about obtaining a medical marijuana licence, the right way? You may be questioning why you should bother obtaining a medical marijuana licence if your local government allows for the sale of recreational marijuana. Why go through the hassle? Having a medical marijuana licence may provide you with several advantages, such as:
1. Access to more CBD-rich cannabis varieties and products.
2. Paying less tax on the purchases you make.
3. Being able to purchase greater quantities at a time.
4. Possibly more leniency should you get caught travelling into a jurisdiction that is less open to cannabis use.

Let's walk through a 3-step process that'll increase your odds of getting approval:
Step #1: Researching.
Often an Internet search of government-sponsored websites will turn up enough information to get you started asking questions. You should be able to find out answers to basic questions as far as which types of individuals have access to cannabis, what needs to be done to obtain authorization, what medical conditions are being covered and how and where can you purchase your medical marijuana.

Once you have an idea as to what ailments are currently being covered under your local government's mandate, you'll be in a better position to make your case with your health care professional. Also, check out local dispensaries and compassion clubs for advice on how to best jump through the approval hoops. Now that you're armed with some solid information about what to do and not do, it's time to find a supportive health-care professional.

Step #2: Finding.
As I see it you have two options before you. You could always go to your current health care professional to make your case for a medical marijuana licence. Or you could find one that is sympathetic to the cause and who has some experience working with patients using medical marijuana.

If your current health care provider has extensive experience with cannabis-related products and an in-depth knowledge of the industry, by all means go to them. Unfortunately, most health care professionals do not have the training nor experience in prescribing medical marijuana. A case in point is that only 1% of doctors in Massachusetts are registered with the state and allowed to prescribe marijuana. Granted you've been able to purchase recreational marijuana in the state since 2016. However, most of this is THC-rich bud, as opposed to CBD-rich products that provide more health benefits in treating a variety of illnesses.

The other option is to seek out a knowledgeable doctor who has a proven track record. To do so, you'll need to do a little investigating. Subtlety asking staff at dispensaries, compassion clubs, or medical marijuana facilities may give you some leads. Ask your pharmacist, close friends, colleagues and family members to suggest potential candidates. At this stage of the game, get some basic contact and background information on each possible advisor. You may even be able to find a doctor being recommended online in a local forum or advocacy group.

Step #3: Selecting.
Once you have a couple of names, set up a meet-and-greet to get a feel for that individual. From your list of good contacts try to touch base by phone to get a preliminary "read" on the individual. If you find that you have made a connection over the phone with someone who may be able to help, then schedule a face-to-face meeting.

When you meet your potential candidate, assess the "outward" appearance of the office, the staff and your doctor in a professional setting. Ideally, you're looking for someone who is a strong role model. Watch and observe how people in the office interact and carry themselves. You can learn a lot about the doctor even before setting foot in his or her office for the meeting.

Before arriving in the office take some time to craft a list of questions that'll enable you to better acquaint yourself with the doctor. You should try to assess the depth of knowledge, wealth of experience and underlying health care philosophy that drives them. Take the time to assess the advisor's familiarity with and ability to discuss and recommend a wide variety of cannabis products. Try to assess if there will be a good personality fit between the two of you. This is critical to establishing a beneficial life-long relationship for you.

Taking the time to find the right individual who is willing to work with you is well worth the time spent. The right individual should be able to steer you in the right direction and hold you accountable for achieving your health care goals.

Before using cannabis, should I consult my physician just the same? Even though CBD-rich cannabis has been shown to improve many health conditions, this is not the case with all ailments or afflictions. Cannabis is a potent drug, capable of producing unwanted side effects, cause significant drug interactions with other medications and be toxic during pregnancy. Granted most of these interactions are with large doses of THC-rich cannabis; however, certain CBD products can also cause negative side effects.

This is why it's so important to find a physician who understands how cannabis works in the body and has a proven track record of prescribing medical marijuana to patients. It's also why you should consult a knowledgeable physician, especially if you have any of these conditions:
1. Auto-immune disorder.
2. Chronic pulmonary disease including bronchitis.
3. Use of blood thinners to treat stroke.
4. Cardio-vascular disease.
5. Mental illness especially schizophrenia and bipolar disease.

Your physician will be able to tell you about those drugs that will either increase or decrease the effects of cannabis. For example, the effects of alcohol typically increase with THC-rich cannabis consumption. Whereas, cannabis decreases or interferes with the herbal antidepressant St. John's Wort.

Should your current physician be unable to give you some concrete answers, ask your local pharmacist. Their knowledge of drug interactions is much more extensive than a typical physician's.

So, what's out there to tantalize my taste buds?

Before we delve into what to buy, here's an overview of the most popular ways that cannabis can be consumed. I've broken them down into three general product categories:

1. Inhalable.
2. Edible.
3. Topical.

But before we delve into the pros and cons of each category of consumption, let's take a quick look at how cannabis can be processed to create a concentrate that can then be used in multiple applications.

Concentrates have several distinct advantages over just dried bud. They are a purer form of cannabis that contains very little vegetative matter. Being concentrated, you'll require less product to create a desired effect. Processing often results in a product that is cleaner and easier to store long-term. Also, concentrates are versatile in that they can be inhaled, ingested or applied to the skin depending on their end use.

When the dried buds are converted into a more concentrated form, this usually involves separating the vegetative matter from the CBD-rich resin that coats the buds and leaves located close to the buds. One simple way to do so, is by dry sifting the buds and "sugar" leaves over a mesh screen that allows the desirable bulbous trichomes to break off the plant matter, pass through the screen and be collected as a dry yellowish product called kief. Under a hand-held microscope, the bulbous trichomes look like clear, white or amber colored mushrooms. This kief can either be pressed to produce hashish or used on its own. Pressing dried kief causes the resinous glands to break and oxidize turning a familiar brown color characteristic of hash.

Another common way of extracting the kief is using a dried ice or regular ice water bath. The buds and leaves are frozen making the trichomes brittle. Then they're placed in mesh bags that trap the vegetative matter but allow the bulbous trichomes to pass through and be collected. Agitating the ice bath slurry breaks off the trichomes.

Kief is not water soluble. It's only soluble in certain oils, fats and alcohol. The ice/water extraction method does a very good job of separating some of the water-soluble, vegetative matter and other organic matter from the wet kief. This wet kief (water hash) can then be dried and added as a base ingredient in virtually any product. I'll be walking you through an easy-to-follow process for making water hash in Section 3 on how to grow your own CBD-rich medicine.

On a commercial scale, both butane and carbon dioxide can be used to produce CBD-rich extracts. Butane gas extraction is currently the most common form of extraction since it's inexpensive to set up, even for the regular Joe. Unfortunately, it's also the most dangerous method as butane gas is explosive.

Carbon dioxide extraction is a safer method of extraction and can produce a cleaner, healthier end product. However, the equipment is costlier and requires extensive training in order to operate. Only large-scale commercial production facilities use this form of extraction technology.

The latest technology making its appearance onto the production scene is the use of a hyperbaric chamber (think scuba diving decompression chamber) for extracting specific cannabinoids.

As you can see, the future of cannabis is in the purification of the raw organic material into clean concentrates that can be used in a variety of applications. Cannabis extracts are easier to ship around the globe and easier to quantify as to cannabinoid and terpene levels when compared to raw bud. Let's explore the pros and cons of each of the three general categories of cannabis consumption before we have you buying any product.

1. Inhalable Products:

The most common means of using cannabis is to either smoke or vape it. The cannabinoids in dried bud, kief, or hash can be converted from their acidic "inactive" form to their decarboxylated "active" form through the mechanics of smoking or vaping. Whether you're smoking or vaping, cannabinoids enter the bloodstream very quickly through the lungs. The effects of your dosing will be felt within minutes.

Since smoking or vaping is a rapid delivery method, you can easily learn how to control your dosage by simply inhaling one dose at a time and waiting two to three minutes between doses. Once you have a base level established, future dosage becomes that much easier to regulate.

Inhalable products can be loosely grouped into three categories, namely smoking, dabbing and vaping.

(a) Smoking:

Smoking cannabis buds is the most common way of getting the cannabinoids into your body. It generally doesn't require any sophisticated equipment, just cigarette paper or a pipe, some crushed bud and a lighter. The downside is that since you're burning the buds, not only do you inhale the cannabinoids but you're also taking in other toxic chemicals, such as hydrogen cyanide, carbon monoxide, tars, and a host of polycyclic aromatic compounds that are known carcinogens. As well, smoking tends to waste a lot more bud compared to other methods of inhalation.

One-hitter cannabis pipes are becoming more popular amongst daily users. These inexpensive, easy-to-use pipes can deliver a controlled dose for those who wish to smoke cannabis to treat their health condition. Should you decide to smoke your cannabis this way, use a light touch and take your time when using a butane lighter. By quickly incinerating the bowl of cannabis with the flame, you end up destroying terpenes and rendering the cannabinoids less effective. Avoid igniting the cannabis with a visible flame. Try to gradually heat the edge of the bowl.

(b) Dabbing:

Dabbing is the process of heating a small quantity of hash or concentrate using a heated "nail" made of titanium, ceramic or quartz along with a water pipe or bong. The "nail" device is usually heated with a butane blowtorch until red hot, then a dab of concentrate is placed on the nail. This flash-melts and boils the concentrate generating a vapor that can be inhaled. Since inhaling the air that's been superheated can burn respiratory tissue, most dabbers cool the vapor through a glass or silicon water pipe.

Most cannabis users shy away from dabbing. They don't care for the elaborate set-up required for traditional dabbing, that of having a dabber, water pipe and blowtorch. For most daily users of cannabis dabbing is not a viable means of self-medicating, especially when out I public. To address this concern, compact handheld units are coming out into the market that use electrical heat to vaporize the concentrate.

The advantage of dabbing is that you can inhale concentrated quantities of cannabinoids with less toxic smoke compared to smoking dried bud. These extracts can reach 80% cannabinoid levels by dry weight, making them extremely potent. Dabbing also delivers cannabinoids into the bloodstream almost instantly. One downside is the facility to overdose on the extract resulting in acute intoxication, which may result in passing out, nausea, or anxiety. Another is the risk of being burned by either the nail, blowtorch or superheated vapor.

(c) Vaporizing:

In 1994, BC Vaporizers coined the name "vaporizer", which is now used to refer to all vaporizer devices in today's market. Vaping is the process of heating dried bud or an extract using a device designed to boil (vaporize) cannabinoids at the optimal temperature for conversion of CBDA (240°F) and THCA (220°F) to CBD and THC. Since the material is not being burned, the harshness and flavor of smoke are absent, along with fewer toxins being inhaled. Vaping gives the user a purer and richer tasting experience.

All vaporizers are composed of three parts. There is an electrical heating element, a bowl-like compartment that holds the cannabis and some way of catching and drawing the vapor up into the lungs, often in the form of a mouthpiece.

Vaporizers fall into two sub-categories, those that primarily use dried bud and kief and those that use cannabis infused oil cartridges or concentrated extracts. Vaporizer pens having an oil or e-juice reservoir are becoming more and more popular with many vape pens being priced under $60 US.

Vaping allows for a more rapid absorption of cannabinoids in the bloodstream. This is why many users report feeling the effects faster than smoking. It's also less of a bronchial irritant than smoking, which can result in a chronic cough developing.

Many vaporizers are compact, discreet and easy to operate in a public setting. This makes vaping an ideal choice for jurisdictions that still frown upon marijuana use.

As with smoking, vaping allows you to make quick adjustments to your dosing since the effects are felt within minutes. Be advised that those vaporizers that use propylene glycol and glycerin may be potentially toxic when they burn. With vaping cartridges being such a new phenomenon, not enough scientific research has been done to prove whether these devices are safe or potentially harmful. Sometimes, it's best to err on the side of caution in these instances.

2. Edible Products:

For the most part, edible products containing cannabinoids are discrete and easy to consume. If you're not comfortable with the idea of smoking or vaping cannabis, edibles are a good alternative. Cannabis can be added to many edible products and beverages. It can be used to make oils and tinctures or packaged in capsules for easy consumption. In the section of the book that deals with how to grow your own medicine, you'll be shown several ways of processing your cannabis to produce an assortment of edible products. Here are the four most common categories of edibles.

(a) Tinctures:

Sublingual alcohol-based tinctures are made by dissolving a cannabis extract in high-proof ethyl alcohol like Everclear. This alcohol-based tincture can be used by placing a drop under the tongue and allowing it to momentarily rest in the mouth to be absorbed sublingually. The effects are typically felt within five minutes, with full effects being felt within twenty minutes. Although not as fast-acting as vaping or smoking, taken sublingually tinctures can be easily dosed.

For those who don't prefer the use or taste of alcohol, glycerin-based tinctures are an option. Glycerin is a sweet-tasting viscous alcohol that's often associated with the "legs" seen sliding down a glass of wine giving the wine some body. Ah wine, helping white men dance.

A major advantage of tinctures is that the terpenes are more effectively delivered by mouth with alcohol-based tinctures, since they are not being heated excessively and vaporized as in smoking. Recall that it is the interplay between cannabinoids and terpenes that is important in the healing process. They also carry none of the harmful chemicals produced by burning and smoking cannabis.

Tinctures are discreet. Most bottles look like homeopathic medicine bottles. Stored in the fridge, they produce no telltale signs of cannabis odours. No need to sneak around to use them with others in your midst.

Also, multiherbal tinctures are coming onto the market. Many herbs can be used with cannabis to create a synergistic effect. For example, passion flower, lemon balm and valerian root induce relaxation and sleep. When combined with a CBD-rich variety, you can induce a more profound state of relaxation.

Not only can tinctures be taken sublingually, they can be added to soups, sauces and gravies just before serving.

The important consideration with tinctures is that they be commercially homogenized otherwise the CBD tends to precipitate out of solution over time. When producing your own tinctures, periodically shaking the solution helps.

27

(b) Cannabis Oil:

When an alcohol-based tincture is slowly heated to evaporate the alcohol, it produces a viscous oil that can also be used sublingually. Known in the industry as Rick Simpson oil, after the Canadian marijuana advocate, this concentrate is an easy way to determine an effective dose. By starting with a drop and increasing one's dosage gradually while monitoring the effects, one can arrive at an effective dose safely without any adverse effects.

(c) Beverages:

Commercially, alcohol-based tinctures can also be added to a variety of alcoholic beverages, whether they be beer, wine, or spirits. One of the world's largest beverage conglomerates, Constellation Brands, has entered into a partnership with Canopy Growth to develop a new line of cannabis-infused alcoholic beverages. Do you think that there might be an investment opportunity there?

Along with the beer and wine industry, soft drink companies are also exploring ways of creating new lines of beverages. You'll soon see energy drinks, health beverages, coffee and tea drinks all being sold in various forms across many jurisdictions as the cannabis industry matures.

(d) Food Products:

Brownies, cookies, gummy bears oh my! The possibilities are endless when it comes to producing cannabis-infused food products. Ingesting cannabis appeals to many novice users as it doesn't require taking up smoking or drinking in order to benefit from the cannabinoids.

The effects of ingesting cannabis generally take thirty to forty-five minutes. This can pose a problem for novice users who'll have one brownie, not feel anything for half an hour and then munch on a second only to have the first brownie kick in. Patience with your dosing is critical. Start low and slow. With experience, you'll be able to determine how your edibles are affecting you.

Also, be aware that the effects of ingesting cannabis are slightly different from inhaling it. Since the cannabis is passing through the digestive tract, a lower percentage of the active ingredients is made readily available by the body. However, the effects can stay longer in the body, which makes it a great choice for nighttime use. Effects typically last four to eight hours depending on the variety, dosage and your personal level of tolerance. This may be just the ticket to getting a restful sleep or going through the workday feeling better.

A disadvantage of eating your medicine is that if you're diabetic or overweight this approach may not be the best option for you when it comes to regular consumption.

Dry cannabis buds can also be used in cooking. Adding a pinch of bud to your favorite recipes at the tail-end of the cooking process can be an effective way of self-medicating. Just ensure that you're not using high heat, which can destroy much of the medicinal benefits. Since cannabis is soluble in oil, it can be added to butter, coconut oil or olive oil to be used as a spread or in salads.

Cannabis extracts can even be dissolved in coconut oil and formed into capsules known as canna-caps. These discreet pills can be taken virtually anywhere. Dosing becomes a lot easier with these handy little capsules. As with other edibles, the effects are usually felt within thirty minutes of ingestion.

3. Topical Products:

Topicals are designed for cannabis extracts to be absorbed directly through the skin. And they're formulated to have a local effect. Most topical products are CBD-rich creams, ointments, oils and salves that are designed to provide relief for conditions such as arthritis, joint and muscle soreness, inflammation, and a myriad of skin conditions.

They typically contain very low doses of THC with most of the cannabinoids coming from CBD-rich plants. Traditionally, Cannabis Sativa (hemp) has been processed on an industrial scale to extract cannabidiol (CBD) for use in topical products. These products can be purchased in most jurisdictions or ordered online. Recently, certain CBD-rich varieties of Cannabis Indica plants grown on an industrial outdoor scale have gained increasing popularity in the production of topicals. This trend is sure to continue as breeders and cultivars develop varieties targeting specific applications.

Cannabis topicals can do a good job of managing localized pain and inflammation since the skin has both CB1 and CB2 receptors that CBD-rich topicals can act on for a therapeutic effect. For those having to take opioids to cope with pain, cannabis topicals can drastically reduce the need to use narcotics or over-the-counter pain medications.

Topicals can vary greatly in how well they deliver cannabinoids and terpenes to an affected area of the body. Most topical applications have dissolved the cannabinoids into lotions and creams that contain glycerine, oil or alcohol. These carriers do a decent job of penetrating the outer layer of the skin.

Anything deeper requires a carrier like DMSO (Dimethyl sulfoxide). DMSO is an industrial solvent that's created as a by-product of paper making. Although DMSO is used world-wide for various health care applications, topicals made with this carrier require some precautionary steps. The main one is keeping any harsh or toxic substances away from the site of application as the carrier will transport these substances deeper into the body.

Always look for topical products that use the purest sources of natural ingredients. Avoid those that contain preservatives like parabens or any artificial fragrances. If you're having a hard time pronouncing the chemical additive in a topical product, it might be a good idea to find one that has simple known ingredients like beeswax, aloe vera, eucalyptus, shea butter or Vitamin E.

The downside of using most commercially available topicals is that cannabinoids don't penetrate the skin very well. If you're suffering from deep tissue or joint pain, inhaling or ingesting cannabinoids often provides better relief. Also, be wary of topical tinctures containing alcohol as they tend to create a burning sensation when applied to open wounds or cracked skin.

Variety is the spice of life.

With literally hundreds of cannabis varieties out in the market, it can be a daunting challenge selecting the right variety to best treat what ails you. Many CBD-rich cannabis varieties can produce dramatic differences in treating certain conditions. These differences are often attributed to the levels of various terpenes and cannabinoids present.

Since the turn of the century, we've seen explosive growth in cannabis breeding programs. Breeders were giving their new creations all sorts of wild and crazy names, like Purple Urkle, Chocolope, or Pirate Radio. The problem with this approach to labeling medicine with "made-up" names, is that you don't know what the chemical breakdown of the main ingredients for that cannabis variety is.

A movement is underfoot by various legal jurisdictions to label cannabis products with "brand" names, based on a chemical profile. Today's technology allows us to genetically and chemically fingerprint each variety of cannabis we come in contact with. This kind of understanding and mapping is necessary if we want to make significant advances in prescribing cannabis varieties for specific ailments or conditions. Although we still do not fully understand the interplay between cannabinoids and terpenoids in producing medicinal effects, advances in international research are finally being shared regularly.

How do I select quality dried cannabis?

The most common cannabis product purchased for recreational and medicinal use is dried bud. CBD-rich buds are initially harvested in any medical cannabis grow operation, at which point they may be processed into a variety of products already outlined above.

The challenge is in selecting which products or what method you would like to pursue for getting those life-giving cannabinoids into your system. Since most users currently smoke, vape or dab cannabis because of its fast delivery, let's take a look at how to select an inhalable product.

Despite our lack of understanding in being able to select cannabis varieties that'll treat certain conditions, all is not lost. The selection process need not be a crap shoot. Here's a four-step approach that'll help you with your cannabis selection:

Step #1: Check out Leafly.com.

One of the largest online databases of cannabis varieties is Leafly.com. The website provides you with a basic understanding of:
1. What each variety is.
2. Where to buy the variety.
3. Its effects and attributes (both positive and negative).
4. The plant's genetics and growing information.
5. Typical flavour profile.
6. Reviews.

This website also has blog posts and videos covering a variety of cannabis-related topics. This is where I do my initial research into various CBD-rich strains available in the market, before I buy. Makes sense, right?

Step #2: Look at the chemical composition on the package.

Pay attention to the chemical breakdown of the cannabinoids and terpenes listed on the packaging of your medicine. Initially, your buying decision will probably be based on what you think (or the dispensary employee thinks) might work best for your particular situation.

Once you do purchase a particular variety, get into the simple habit of logging your purchases in a notebook or spreadsheet over time. Record any chemical analysis notes and the physiological effects that each variety produces. It is through this sort of collective wisdom that you'll be able to narrow down your choices to those cultivars that give you the biggest bang for your buck.

Step #3: Smell the aroma.

Bud aroma is often a good indicator of what the medicinal properties of a cannabis variety might be. Cannabis contains volatile terpenes that give it distinctive aromas. The scent of pine (Pinene) is often associated with varieties that have a stimulating, uplifting effect. Plants with a citrus aroma (Limonene) often create a sense of euphoria helping to combat depression. Plants smelling of lavender (Linalool) and grape (Myrcene) are known to produce more relaxing or sedative effects.

Cannabis that smells of green grass or has a strong vegetative smell has not been cured properly and should be avoided. The same can be said of cannabis that has little aroma. It may be too old or was exposed to excessive heat that drove off many of the terpenes. Terpenes work synergistically with cannabinoids to produce certain desirable health benefits. Odorless cannabis may still be potent with cannabinoids, but you lose some of the medicinal benefits. Over time, as you learn how to associate aroma with effects, you'll become more adept in selecting over-the-counter varieties that'll best meet your needs.

Here in a nutshell are some of the most important terpenes that are present in significant quantities in many varieties of cannabis along with some of the known benefits:
1. Myrcene: muscle relaxant, sedative, analgesic, antioxidant
2. Pinene: aids short-term memory, antibiotic, anti-inflammatory
3. Limonene: anti-depressant, sedative, anti-inflammatory, anti-tumor
4. Linalool: calming, anti-anxiety, anesthetic
5. Caryophyllene: anti-inflammatory, analgesic, cytoprotective
6. Terpinolene: cognitive clarity, antidepressant, anti-anxiety
7. Cineole (eucalyptol): anti-inflammatory, antiviral, antibiotic, anti-depressant.

Step #4: Examine the buds closely.

Using a magnifying lens or hand-held microscope, do a visual inspection of the buds under natural sunlight if possible. Natural sunlight is better than fluorescents in that you'll be able to see discolorations easier. The buds should range in color from light to dark green. You may also see yellow or red coloration patterns depending on the variety. Odd discoloration or excessive browning often indicates that the cannabis is of an inferior quality.

Look for large, intact bulbous trichomes. The more of them, the better the quality of the bud. The trichomes should be clear to milky in appearance. Avoid buds with trichomes that have excessive amber coloring. This usually indicates that the plants were harvested after their peak period of cannabinoid production.

Use your magnifying lens to check for pest infestations, such as gnats, mites or aphids that have been trapped by the sticky trichome resin. Also look for signs of mildew and mold that typically show up as white or grey deposits or fuzz on any "sugar" leaves close to the buds.

Which CBD-rich varieties are the best to use?

Before I touch on this topic, it might be helpful to illustrate how the cannabis industry is evolving and what to expect in the future as to the types and quality of the medicine being produced.

Currently, a high percentage of CBD is being derived from hemp, which is characteristically low in THC and higher in CBD concentrations. Industrial hemp is being grown in many countries around the world for its CBD content, with some amount being produced in select States in America. Large volumes of hemp need to be processed in order to extract enough CBD to be processed into various medicinal products.

However, where the real benefits for consumers is going to come from is in the production and processing of CBD-rich cannabis varieties. This is currently the trend in Canada, which is poised to take on a dominant role in the production of CBD-based extracts. Current and future research into the interplay between CBD (along with its derivatives) and terpenes found in cannabis cultivars opens up more medicinal product options than hemp plants alone.

Advances in the breeding and cultivation of cannabis have resulted in a plethora of varieties being available on the market. So, which ones offer the most promise?

Not knowing your particular medical condition or history, it would be foolish of me to recommend certain strains. However, what I can offer is an overview of some of the more widely-used varieties that have shown promise in treating a number of ailments.

I'll share with you some background knowledge about:
1. the genetics behind each variety,
2. the average ratios and levels of CBD and THC present,
3. the key terpenes present (if known), and
4. the indoor growing expectations and yield.

If you're considering growing your own medicine in the future, these collective insights should help you with seed or clone selection down the road. You'll gain some in depth knowledge on this topic in the next section on how to set up a discrete closet grow. In the meantime, let's uncork these numbers and let them breathe, like a good bottle of French Bordeaux wine.

Here are ten CBD-rich varieties to consider investigating for your personal use:

1. Cannatonic

Cannatonic was developed by Resin Seeds out of Spain in 2008 and is a cross between Reina Madre and New York City Diesel. It was the strain that started the CBD revolution. The Cannatonic family includes varieties such as AC/DC, Dancehall and Ringo's Gift.

It often produces up to 17% CBD with 6% THC. Cannatonic typically produces average CBD to THC ratios around 2:1, which means that users can benefit from the synergistic relationship between the various cannabinoids present. As you can see, it develops a significant amount of CBD; however, there are many strains out there that produce higher CBD-levels.

The buds produce terpene aromas of citrus and pine.

This strain is best-suited for growers who have some experience. It's quite a short plant that can be successfully grown indoors, outdoors, or in greenhouse operations with a 9 to 10-week flowering period. Grown indoors under ideal conditions the yield will be moderate to high. It can produce 3 to 6 oz/ft^2 of caramel-colored CBD-rich buds or 24 to 48 oz. in a 2' x 4' closet grow.

It's known for its ability to relax the body without the couch-lock effect. Cannatonic is often used to relieve pain, anxiety, muscle spasms and migraines while maintaining your energy level.

2. AC/DC

AC/DC is a high CBD strain with low THC levels. It is a derivative of Cannatonic that produces average CBD to THC ratios of 20:1. CBD levels are typically between 16% and 24%.

Having a high CBD ratio makes this a favorite with those looking for a daily medicinal cannabis strain that'll relieve tension, pain and anxiety without any psychoactive effects. It can provide a certain degree of alertness, focus and mental clarity.

Myrcene terpene levels tend to be high with this plant, especially when grown outdoors in full sun. It also has significant levels of Linalool, Limonene and Caryophyllene. It is easily grown outdoors but tends to be a bit more challenging for indoor growth. Being a high CBD variety, it's sensitive to overfeeding. Grown indoors it'll reach average heights of 36" to 48". AC/DC flowers quickly within a 7 to 8-week period. It produces a moderate yield of 1 to 3 oz/ft^2 of CBD-rich buds or 8 to 24 oz. in a 2' x 4' closet grow.

AC/DC is often used to treat pain, anxiety, chemotherapy side effects and epilepsy.

3. Charlotte's Web

Here's another high CBD variety with very low THC levels. Charlotte's Web produces an average ratio of 20:1 with CBD concentrations between 17% and 20%. THC levels are below 0.5%.

Developed by the Colorado-based Stanley Brothers in 2013, Charlotte's Web was successfully used to treat Charlotte Fiji's Dravet Syndrome so that her daily seizures became more manageable. It became the focus of national attention for making medical cannabis legally accessible for epileptic patients across the United States.

Being a hemp-derived product from Cannabis Sativa plants, the seeds of this particular CBD-rich variety are not available commercially (as of publication).

It has an earthy or woody fragrance with some hints of lemon and light floral scents.
The flavor profile is a combination of pine, sage and citrus.

This particular variety of CBD-rich cannabis is mentioned here because of its widespread use to treat younger patients with Dravet syndrome, epilepsy, and the negative effects of traditional cancer treatments.

It has been known to provide relief for chronic pain, fibromyalgia and Parkinson's disease symptoms.

4. Harlequin

Harlequin is a descendent of Columbian Gold cannabis, a Nepali Indica variety, and Thai and Swiss landrace varieties. It usually develops a CBD:THC ratio of 5:2 with typical CBD levels of 8% to 16% and low THC levels of 4% to 7%.

Harlequin is an easy plant to grow indoors with big yields. It flowers in just 7 to 9 weeks, but it tends to stretch to a height of 5 or 6 feet if not trained to grow out rather than up. It often produces 3 to 6 oz/ft^2 of CBD-rich buds or 24 to 48 oz. in a 2' x 4' closet grow.

Predominant flavors of Harlequin are earthy, sweet and flowery. The most prominent terpenes are pinene, myrcene and caryophyllene.

Harlequin is known for its long-lasting ability to treat pain and anxiety. CBD and THC working together are a very effective analgesic. It also allows the body to relax without sedation. The CBD present in this variety makes it a good anti-inflammatory choice.

5. Pennywise

Pennywise was created by TGA Subcool Seeds by crossing Harlequin with Jack the Ripper. It typically displays a CBD:THC ratio of 1:1 with CBD levels in the range of 12% to 15%.

Known for its sweet aroma and notes of coffee and spice, it has sweet flavors of bubble gum, spice and herbs.

Pennywise is easy to grow indoors, flowering in 8 to 9 weeks, with a medium height of 3 to 4 feet. It also produces a moderate yield of 1 to 3 oz/ft^2 of CBD-rich buds or 8 to 24 oz. in a 2' x 4' closet grow.

This variety is often recommended for daytime users to relax. It has been helpful for treating PTSD, epilepsy, anxiety attacks, and the effects of cancer treatments.

6. Harle-Tsu

Harle-Tsu was bred by Southern Humboldt Seed Collective by crossing Harlequin with Sour Tsunami. It's big in the CBD department with typical levels of 20% to 24% and a high 20:1 ratio of CBD to THC.

Harle-Tsu has spicy, herbal and pine aromas. Sweet citrus and woody flavors predominate on the taste buds along with some peppery notes.

Indoors the plant with flower in 8 weeks, growing to an average height of 36" to 48" making it easy to train. Like Harlequin, it produces a moderate yield of 1 to 3 oz/ft^2 of CBD-rich buds or 8 to 24 oz. in a 2' x 4' closet grow.

Harle-Tsu provides stress, pain and inflammation relief without producing a psychoactive high. This is a great variety for daytime use, especially in combatting depression.

7. Ringo's Gift

Taking Harle-Tsu to the next level, Ringo's gift crosses Harle-Tsu with AC/DC. This strain was named after CBD pioneer, Lawrence Ringo who founded Southern Humboldt Seed Collective.

Like Harle-Tsu, it has a high CBD:THC ratio of 20:1. It produces an average CBD level of 15% with very low THC levels under 1%.

On the palate it is sweet, floral, and earthy with some spicy hints of mint.

Ringo's Gift is moderately difficult to grow indoors, attaining heights of 36" to 48", which requires that it be trained for small grow spaces. Like its parent plant AC/DC, Ringo's Gift produces average indoor yields of 1 to 3 oz/ft^2 of CBD-rich buds or 8 to 24 oz. in a 2' x 4' closet grow.

You can expect a full body relaxation, but without the couch-lock effect. Ringo's Gift is popular to better cope with chronic pain, anxiety, panic attacks, arthritis, PTSD, and muscle spasms.

---

8. CBD Therapy

Here's another CBD-rich variety with average CBD:THC ratios of 20:1, along with CBD concentrations of 8% to 10% and very low THC levels under 0.5%.

This varietal was created by CBD Crew seedbank. CBD Crew is an international collaboration project of 3 breeders dedicated to producing a line of CBD-rich cannabis varieties.

It has a sweet, fruity tropical taste with an earthy aroma.

Like many of the CBD-rich varieties presented thus far, CBD Therapy grows to a moderate height and flowers within an 8 to 9-week period. It has moderate indoor yields of 1 to 3 oz/ft^2, which equates to 8 to 24 oz. in a 2' x 4' closet grow.

The body-centred effects of CBD Therapy invoke calming and relaxing feelings.

It is often used for fibromyalgia, Crohn's, epilepsy, Dravet syndrome, and inflammation.

9. CBD OG

CBD OG is a cross between Lion's Tabernacle and SFV OG. It has a higher level of THC with typical CBD:THC ratios of 1:1 and CBD levels between 5% and 10%. Since it does have an appreciable level of THC, CBD OG produces a moderate cerebral high.

This cannabis variety has produced by Cali Connection from California and won the Best CBD Flower at the 2015 Cannabis Cup.

CBD OG produces intense lemon, oil and spicy notes.

It's a compact plant that's easy to grow indoors with flowering times of 8 to 9 weeks and produces average yields.

CBD OG is often recommended for tension, pain, and anxiety.

---

10. Sour Tsunami

Sour Tsunami was created by Lawrence Ringo of Southern Humboldt Seed Collective, by crossing Sour Diesel with NYC Diesel. It offers an equal ratio of CBD with THC producing a light psychoactive effect. CBD levels are typically around 11%.

Sour Tsunami displays aromas of citrus and wood, along with flavors of sour, citrus and pine.

This plant can be difficult to grow indoors as it tends to stretch to 6 feet when given the opportunity. Therefore, it needs to be trained for a closet grow. Normal flowering occurs in 8 to 9 weeks. It produces a moderate yield of 2 to 4 oz/ft^2 of CBD-rich buds or 16 to 32 oz. in a 2' x 4' closet grow.

Sour Tsunami is often prescribed for daytime use, to help relieve pain, tension, and anxiety, while pleasantly uplifting the mood.

Now that you have an idea as to some of the more popular CBD-rich varieties out in the market, let's look at what ailments CBD does help based on recent anecdotal evidence and current scientific research.

Chapter 3: What Ailments Does CBD Help?

Can cannabis cure disease?

No. Despite the hype out in the market that cannabis is a cure for cancer or other ailments, this has not been scientifically proven to be the case. Yes, cannabis can help better manage and cope with various ailments, but it's not a definitive cure for disease.

If you're looking at a one-step cure for what ails you, you're adopting the wrong approach. Your overall health is determined by a number of factors. Physical fitness, mental health, nutrition and sleeping habits all play a factor in your overall health. To think that one approach is going to miraculously heal you of what health challenge you may currently be faced with, is not the path to wellness.

I'm not going to pee on your leg and tell you it's raining. It can be challenging and confusing trying to figure out what does and doesn't work for coping with illness.

So, how do you get the most benefit from using any cannabis product? The most direct answer? By using a multi-faceted approach to health care and wellness, your chances of success increase tenfold. More on this in a moment.

For which common ailments can CBD-rich cannabis have a positive effect? It's unfortunate that cannabis is not the be all and end all of medical treatments for what ails us. However, both CBD and THC offer the user health benefits that have been documented anecdotally (through observations) and scientifically (through limited research). Let's explore twenty-five specific ailments with which CBD-rich cannabis has shown to help individuals better cope or treat what ails them.

Just as a side note, I'll cover specific dosing recommendations for various ways of ingesting CBD products in the next chapter that addresses specifically how to use cannabis products.

———

Twenty-five ailments that CBD helps:

1. Acne:

Acne is the most common skin disease across the globe. It's caused by the proliferation of sebocytes in the sebaceous glands that die, clogging the glands and inviting bacterial growth to occur. CBD has been shown to regulate this proliferation. Coupled with the terpenes Limonene or Caryophyllene, it's also effective against inflammation.

Topical CBD in high concentrations has been shown to be an effective anti-acne treatment. It can also treat a wide range of skin disorders, such as eczema and dermatitis.

When choosing a topical ointment or cream, select one with a high concentration of CBD. Cannabinoids have a hard time penetrating the skin when applied topically and may need some warmth, friction and a higher dosage to provide adequate absorption.

2. ALS (Amyotrophic Lateral Sclerosis) Syndrome:

ALS is the progressive loss of muscle strength that often leads to death from respiratory failure and weight loss. CBD has been shown to be moderately effective in reducing certain symptoms, like pain, depression, drooling and appetite loss.

Higher doses of CBD combined with a small amount of THC seems to work best. Up to 300 mg of oral CBD per day, along with low doses of 3.5 to 5.0 mg of THC taken twice daily has shown promise. Look for cannabis varieties containing the terpene Caryophyllene, which is a potent neuroprotector and anti-inflammatory. High Caryophyllene varieties like Cookies or Kryptonite can be combined with high CBD cultivars to arrive at an appropriate combination.

3. Anxiety Disorder:

Anxiety is the unpleasant sensation of apprehension when confronted with an unknown or fear-inducing situation. Cannabis has been used for thousands of years to treat anxiety. Next to pain, anxiety is one of the most frequent reasons why individuals take cannabis.

However, those cannabis varieties high in THC can trigger anxiety and paranoia for some individuals. If you're going to treat your anxiety with cannabis, CBD-rich varieties may be the best choice or low-dose THC ones. It appears that social anxiety and panic disorders can be more effectively treated with CBD than THC.

Look for CBD-rich varieties that are high in the terpenes Limonene or Linalool, which have been shown to have antidepressant and calming properties.

Doses between 2.5 and 10 mg of CBD can be well-tolerated by most users. THC dosage should be kept low at levels between 1 and 3 mg.

Since a fast-acting method of delivery is preferred with those suffering from "panic" or anxiety attacks, using a spray or taking cannabinoids sublingually is recommended, as is smoking or vaping. Look for products or varietals having a CDB:THC ratio greater than 10:1. As mentioned, also seek out varieties high in limonene or linalool. Both these terpenes are known for their calming effects.

4. Arthritis:

Both rheumatoid and osteoarthritis can be treated with cannabinoids. Rheumatoid arthritis is an autoimmune disease that typically causes severe joint pain and damage, resulting in disability. Osteoarthritis affects the bones. It often causes cartilage loss in the spine, hips and knees.

When CBD and THC work synergistically together, they provide a positive anti-inflammatory response, along with a reduction in joint pain often associated with this condition. Although THC on its own reduces severe chronic pain, most arthritic individuals benefit from a combination of both types of cannabinoids. This is especially so for older patients who have had limited exposure to THC and its psychoactive properties. One option to consider is combining a THC strain like Trainwreck or Animal Cookies with a CBD strain like AC/DC or Cannatonic to produce the desired effect.

It may be advisable to look for CBD-rich cannabis strains that also have a significant amount of THC when looking at combining pain management with reducing joint inflammation. Also, look for varieties containing terpenes like Myrcene, Limonene, and Linalool, which may add some additional synergistic effects.

Begin with low doses (2.5 to 5.0 mg) of an ingestible product so that you may benefit from the long-lasting effects of the cannabinoids. Although smoking or vaping cannabis is an option, those with balance issues should err on the side of caution by inhaling very small doses to start.

If you decide to use a topical ointment for joint relief, look for formulations that contain decarboxylated CBD/THC. The decarboxylated form of CBD or THC is the active form of the cannabinoids. Be advised that CBD and especially THC are poorly absorbed through the skin. To enhance the effectiveness of a topical application, gently massage and warm the ointment at the joint site.

5. Asthma:

Asthma is a common respiratory ailment. It's an inflammatory condition of the air passages whereby the individual experiences obstruction of the airway or bronchospasm.

It is well known that THC can elicit a strong bronchodilation effect, which you would think would help relieve some of the symptoms of asthma. For light cannabis smokers minimal damage of the lungs occurs. However, heavy smokers often develop bronchitis, since smoking cannabis is similar to smoking the toxins associated with tobacco.

Recent research has shown that smoking or vaping CBD-rich varieties can be effective in treating inflammatory lung diseases and helps to regulate the inflammatory response in asthma.

Given the choice, vape any cannabis as opposed to smoking. Since asthma can be exasperated by some of the toxins found in smoking, vaping is a safer alternative.

Extremely small doses of THC are all that is required to treat bronchospasm. Doses in the neighborhood of 200 mcg have proven to be effective. By combining THC with CBD, you may be getting a better anti-inflammatory response than with THC alone. CBD doses between 10 mg and 20 mg may prove to be effective.

Look for cannabis strains like Pinene Kush, Blue Dream, Purple Urkle or Grape Ape that are high in Pinene, as this is a known bronchodilator.

6. Autism:

Autism is a complex neurobehavioral condition, often characterized by impaired communication and social interaction.

Unfortunately, little has been published as to the merits of CBD as a potential treatment for autism spectrum symptoms. Recent studies in Israel that involve treating children with CBD have been showing promise. It may be that cannabidiol could be a better option in the future for helping to improve social interactions and calm repetitive behaviours, as opposed to our current potent medication approach.

As for dosage for the use of CBD-rich products for better managing autism, consult with a local health care professional who is up-to-date with the current research into the benefits of cannabinoids for autism. I would love to be able to provide you with some concrete guidelines as to the benefits of CBD use for the treatment of autism, but unfortunately research is still in its infancy.

Should you be looking for an intermediary solution in the meantime, consider exploring ingestible products as opposed to inhaled ones. As well, look for CBD varieties high in the terpenes Myrcene and Linalool, which are known for their calming and anti-anxiety effects.

7. Bipolar Disorder:

Bipolar is a mood disorder that has the individual experiencing recurring episodes of depression and mania, with depression being the most common symptom. Cannabis has shown to help relieve the anxiety often seen after a bout of depression or mania. It may also show promise in relieving other symptoms of bipolar disorder that are often treated with heavy pharmaceuticals prescribed by a psychiatrist.

Choose high CBD to THC ratio cannabis varieties having a ratio above 10:1. You'll receive the anti-anxiety effect, while reducing the psycho-activity. CBD doses of 2.5 mg to 5.0 mg taken a few times during the day have shown positive effects in reducing anxiety. The terpene Limonene can produce an uplifting effect, which may help with symptoms of depression. Linalool has been shown to help induce a calming effect, along with Myrcene.

For faster relief, consider using vaped or smoked products to relieve anxiety associated with bipolar disorder. Ingestion of CBD-rich cannabis products is also an option but has a slower response time for reducing anxiety levels.

8. Cancer:

Cancer is a condition where there is abnormal cell growth causing healthy tissue to be destroyed. Cannabis is not a cure for cancer. Cannabis should not replace current methods of treatment for cancer. Nor, should cannabis be used to help treat "all" forms of cancer. However, it can be used to help with the patient's overall condition, improving one's quality of life.

Cannabis has been shown to help address many negative symptoms associated with cancer, such as pain, insomnia, medical treatment nausea, weight loss and appetite. Varieties that contain a blend of CBD and THC often show better results than taking either cannabinoid on its own. And blended varieties are effective in improving the quality of life by helping recently-diagnosed individuals better cope with feelings of anxiety or depression.

Unfortunately, not enough clinical research has been done to look at cannabis as being an effective treatment for cancer. However, it does show promise as an antitumor medication in killing certain types of cancer cells.

The Canadian cannabis advocate Rick Simpson, creator of Rick Simpson oil or Phoenix Tears, has a strong following of cancer patients looking for ways to improve the quality of their lives while fighting cancer. You'll learn about making quality Rick Simpson oil in the section of the book that explores how to grow and produce your own CBD-rich medicine.

Depending on the specific negative symptom(s) you're looking at reducing (i.e. pain, nausea, appetite, anxiety, etc.), this will dictate the dosage of cannabinoids to take.

One of the most effective methods of ingestion is sublingually in an oil form, which allows the cancer patient to gauge the effects of taking a dose and being able to accurately titrate the correct concentrated dosage.

An alternative is the ingestion of an edible product or capsule that'll have longer-lasting effects, but it must be taken 1 to 2 hours before the onset of the symptoms, such as just before a chemo-therapy session.

Vaporization or smoking cannabis is effective for certain types of symptoms as its effects are felt almost immediately making it easy to adjust one's personal dosage.

Your best bet is to look at what specific symptoms you would like to reduce in order of priority, then look into the dosing recommendations for each of those conditions.

9. Chronic Fatigue Syndrome:

Chronic fatigue syndrome (CFS) is a persistence of symptoms like fatigue, insomnia, pain, sore throat, headaches or loss of concentration over at least a 6-month period of time with these symptoms occurring at the time of the onset of the syndrome.

Chronic fatigue syndrome is little understood and peer-reviewed research studies looking into the use of cannabinoids to help treat it almost non-existent.

CBD-rich varieties have the potential to reduce many of the negative symptoms associated with CFS. Consider using varieties with at least a 3 to1 ratio of CBD to THC in order to better collectively address many of the symptoms. Doses of 25 mg to 40 mg can be tolerated by many sufferers.

Sub-lingual ingestion of an oil or tincture is the preferred method of absorption, with vaping or smoking CBD-rich strains as an alternative method.

10. Depression:

Depression is a mood disorder accompanied by feeling of sadness, along with loss of interest or motivation.

Severe forms of depression such as major depressive disorder (MDD) or depressed mood (DM) are best treated with current, conventional antidepressants. Where cannabis and specifically CBD offers help is with mood elevation and anxiety relief. This is often seen when a patient has just been given a medical diagnosis or during treatment regimes.

CBD varieties high in the terpenes Limonene and Linalool have shown promise in acting as an antidepressant. Light doses of 5 mg to 10 mg of CBD taken during the day are often recommended for symptoms of anxiety. Look for a ratio of CBD:THC of 10:1 or higher.

Taking CBD either sublingually, smoked or vaped is a fast-acting means of delivering the medicine. These methods of ingestion are also easy approaches for gauging dosage. I should also mention that If you're new to smoking or vaping flowers, always start with a match-head size dose. Small doses are easier to titrate on an individual basis.

11. Diabetes:

Diabetes is a disease in which insulin production by the pancreas is impaired resulting in elevated blood glucose levels leading to heart disease, blindness, kidney disease, stroke and other tissue damage.

Type 1 diabetes is typically seen with children and young adults who are unable to produce insulin. Whereas Type 2 diabetes, or onset diabetes often occurs in adults suffering from obesity and poor eating choices. This is the most common form of diabetes.

Recent research is pointing to the use of the non-psychoactive cannabinoids CBD, CBDV and THCV for helping the pancreas regulate insulin levels. Research is still in its infancy when it comes to determining the effectiveness of certain cannabinoids in treating diabetes. More research is needed for assessing the proper dosage of the three promising cannabinoids mentioned. And both oral and vaporized use of these particular cannabinoids is currently being explored.

12. Drug Addiction:

Drug addiction to painkillers is a growing concern in the medical community, as is stimulant abuse.

CBD taken alongside opioid painkillers has shown promise in reducing the quantity of opioid medication required for pain relief. This translates into fewer opioids being prescribed and shorter treatment plans being set up, which ultimately reduces the risk of opioid addiction. CBD has also shown to reduce tobacco dependency in chronic users.

Look for CBD/THC varieties containing low levels of Myrcene, but high levels of Caryophyllene with a CBD:THC ratio around 1:1. For chronic pain relief, THC dominant varieties may prove to be a better alternative. However, using cannabis strains containing both major cannabinoids decreases the risk of "problem cannabis" arising when using high-THC products alone. Problem cannabis is the dependency of using THC-rich cannabis in excess on a daily basis as tolerance requires increased dosing to achieve the same effect.

Both oral and inhaled ingestion methods can be effective means of addressing drug addiction. Begin by establishing the lowest effective dose that'll provide pain relief in conjunction with your painkillers. A dosage of 2.5 mg to 5 mg is often recommended to start.

13. Fibromyalgia:

Fibromyalgia is a chronic disorder characterized by widespread musculoskeletal pain accompanied by fatigue, sleep, memory and mood issues. It is thought that fibromyalgia amplifies sensations of pain by affecting how your brain processes pain signals.

Cannabis has been shown to reduce stiffness, increase relaxation, improve sleep, and reduce pain in sufferers of fibromyalgia. Cannabis can be more effective in the treatment of fibromyalgia than current pharmaceutical options out in the market.

CBD doses ranging from 4 mg to 15 mg have been reported by some patients to be effective. Also, look for cannabis varieties that also have some THC in a CBD:THC ratio around 2:1. A popular varietal to consider using is Harlequin. An initial dose of 5 mg CBD to 2.5 mg THC is recommended.

Oral ingestion of CBD-rich cannabis products provides longer-lasting relief than vaping or smoking. Given the choice, vaporization is a better option than smoking, since some of the combustible by-products can increase inflammation. The exact opposite of one's desired outcome.

14. Gastrointestinal Disorders:

A myriad of gastro-intestinal disorders exist. Unfortunately, not all disorders benefit from the use of CBD-rich cultivars. For example, appetite stimulation may best be achieved with low doses of THC as opposed to CBD. And THC varieties containing the terpene Caryophyllene help individuals better cope with diarrhea.

If constipation or inflammation along the GI tract are symptoms you're experiencing, then CBD-rich varieties can calm gut inflammation and increase motility. For gut pain a combination of CBD and THC with high Myrcene levels may help.

When properly formulated, oral cannabis concentrates can be very soothing for the GI tract. And both vaping and smoking have the advantage of providing quick relief.

Dosage is condition dependent. For constipation challenges, begin with low doses of 2.5 mg to 5 mg of CBD and increase your dosage slowly to find the lowest possible effective dose.

15. Glaucoma:

Glaucoma is an eye disease where the optic nerve is damaged by elevated ocular pressure. This often leads to loss of central vision and blindness. It is the most common type of irreversible blindness in the world.

Both CBD and THC provide neuro-protective benefits. However, high-CBD varieties offer more potential neuro-protective effect on the optic nerve than THC. Consider trying varieties having a CBD:THC ratio greater than 10:1 in order to optimize the effect.

Oral ingestion is the preferred method of delivery because of its long-lasting effects. Taking a dose of 5 mg once in the morning and then later in the afternoon may provide long-term benefits. CBD concentrates could also be sprayed or taken sublingually for faster absorption. Unfortunately, no safe and effective eye drop medication containing CBD has been formulated as of this writing. A topical eye-drop application may prove to be an optimal method of administration. Time will tell.

16. Insomnia:

Insomnia is a psychological condition where an individual has trouble falling asleep or staying asleep at night. The most common treatment is sleep medication. However, inroads are being made into the dosage and delivery of cannabinoids as an effective more natural alternative.

THC alone has been shown to induce sleep, whereas CBD alone tends to promote wakefulness. However, CBD helps to reduce anxiety, which is a major cause of insomnia. Taking CBD in combination with THC makes it easier for an individual to fall asleep initially. The sedative effects of taking THC will often kick in 60 to 90 minutes after initial dosing.

The major key to sleep management is proper sleep hygiene, which allows your body and mind to transition quickly into a resting state. Exposure to bright lights, especially TV's or computers and disruption from noises should be reduced at least 30 minutes prior to bedtime.

Along with this, consider using a non-psycho-active CBD-rich concentrate that could be taken sublingually periodically throughout the day to reduce your stress level. This may be the most effective approach to use when combined with good sleep hygiene. CBD dosage should be around 5 mg per application and adjusted upward as needed to find an effective dosage.

An alternative to try is to orally take a CBD:THC variety about an hour before bedtime, which may provide a longer-lasting sleep effect. THC recommended for sleep is often prescribed at a dosing level of 5 mg to 7.5 mg at least an hour before lights out. In general, look for cannabis varieties that are high in the terpenes Linalool and Myrcene.

17. Nausea:

Nausea is an intense feeling of sickness with an inclination to vomit. Both acute and anticipatory nausea can be treated with cannabis. Acute nausea is often associated with a negative reaction to medications, especially opioids. Whereas anticipatory nausea is triggered by traumatic memories or fears.

CBD has been shown to help patients suffering from acute nausea as it tends to reduce overall anxiety. It also has therapeutic benefits for anticipatory nausea. But what is more encouraging is that CBDA may prove to be a more effective solution for treating anticipatory nausea than any known treatments thus far.

Should you be pregnant or nursing, the use of cannabis medicines to treat nausea should be avoided, especially those containing significant levels of THC.

As you know, orally ingested CBD products and sublingual concentrates can be effective in providing long-lasting relief. Ideally, CBDA concentrates should be sought out when they do hit the market as they show promise as being a potent anti-nausea compound.

THC is often prescribed in doses of 2.5 mg to 10 mg to combat nausea associated with chemotherapy. CBD is typically recommended as a supplement to taking THC during the daytime in 5 mg doses. For both cannabinoids, avoid varieties high in Pinene as this terpene may actually increase the onset of anticipatory nausea by supporting the generation of negative memories.

18. Neuropathy:

Neuropathy is a disease or dysfunction of the peripheral nerves, characterized by pain or numbness in the back, face, hands, thighs or feet. Diabetes is the most common cause.

Chemotherapy-induced neuropathy seems to be more effectively treated with CBD or a CBD:THC variety than a THC cultivar alone. Whereas, cancer-related pain seems to be more effectively controlled with THC alone.

Low to moderate doses of cannabinoids are typically prescribed for neuropathic pain.

Inhalation of cannabis either by vaping or smoking is the preferred method for pain management due to neuropathy. Relief can be experienced within a few minutes of ingestion. Alternatively, cannabis concentrates taken sublingually can provide relief within a 20-minute window. For longer-lasting relief of up to 6 hours, an edible product could be selected.

High concentration topical salves may also be experimented with for localized pain. Since cannabinoids are poorly absorbed through the skin, higher concentrations may be required in order to benefit from a topical application.

Choose between high-CBD cultivars or varieties having a CBD:THC ratio at least 1:1 like Harlequin (5:2), which has been shown to be effective. CBD-rich varieties with CBD:THC ratios of 20:1 also show promise in providing anti-inflammatory properties that contribute to neuropathic pain.

And look for cannabis varieties high in the terpene Caryophyllene, which is known for its anti-inflammatory qualities.

19. Pain:

One of the most common conditions whereby cannabis is prescribed by health care professionals is pain. Pain comes in all shapes and sizes. It is well-known that THC can reduce pain symptoms, but what about CBD and its derivatives?

CBD taken in conjunction with THC seems to provide the right level of pain relief with fewer negative side effects. The key to pain management is finding the lowest effective dose, as higher doses of cannabinoids may actually contribute to the onset of pain or in the case of THC cause intoxication.

When taken orally, CBD prolongs the effects of THC while reducing some of the negative side effects. A CBD:THC ratio of 1:1 is often prescribed in low to moderate doses of 2.5 mg to 5 mg of each cannabinoid. Adjusting these dosing factors to find your particular sweet spot for relief requires some patience and experimentation.

Although vaporization and smoking provide faster relief, caution needs to be exercised in determining the minimal effective dose. Starting with a match-stick size flower and waiting 20 to 30 minutes to assess the desired effects is a prudent approach.

CBD-rich topical applications can be effective in relieving pain associated with skin inflammation disorders. For topical applications to work effectively the pain must be localized at a particular joint or peripheral nerve.

Look for cannabis cultivars high in the terpene Myrcene, a known analgesic with sedating properties. Caryophyllene in CBD-rich varieties also provides anti-inflammatory effects.

20. Palliative Care:

Palliative care is a multidisciplinary approach to providing medical care for people with life-limiting illnesses. Cannabis can help provide relief for certain types of pain, physical distress and mental stress associated with quality-of-life issues.

CBD helps to ease physical and mental distress, while THC provides pain relief. Stress-related anxiety that is often seen in terminally ill patients can be reduced with CBD. Its use throughout the day can allow these patients to experience more restorative sleep and reduce mental stress levels thus improving the quality of end of life. In essence CBD can help reduce suffering in terminally ill patients.

Oral ingestion of 10 to 15 mg of a CBD-rich cultivar is the preferred method of application, since most health care facilities prohibit smoking or vaping on site. This can be done twice a day in order to provide the benefits of cannabis over the course of a 10 to 12-hour block of time.

21. Pediatric Epilepsy:

Pediatric epilepsy occurs in young patients who experience recurring epileptic seizures. It's a neurological disorder that causes seizures or unusual behaviours and is often treated with pharmaceuticals.

Although THC use amongst children is strongly ill advised, CBD may prove to be an effective means of helping children cope with epileptic seizures better than conventional therapies and drugs. More research needs to be done in this regard.

High-CBD varieties have been shown to be effective in reducing the frequency and severity of seizures in many children.

Sublingual ingestion of a CBD-rich oil or tincture is the preferred method of delivery as the effects can be seen relatively quickly. Since each case is unique, a general dosing recommendation would be difficult to propose. Your best bet is to start with a small oral dose, wait 20 to 30 minutes to assess the degree of effectiveness and adjust the dosing accordingly.

22. Post-Traumatic Stress Disorder (PTSD):

Post-traumatic stress disorder develops in individuals who have been exposed to extreme traumatic stress that involves direct exposure to harm or death. It's often seen with returning war veterans. In the 60's, an estimated 50% of returning Vietnam veterans used cannabis to cope with this disorder and the stresses of war.

CBD has shown to be an effective treatment in reducing the memories that trigger the onset of the negative symptoms associated with post-traumatic stress. CBD could be another effective weapon along with cognitive behaviour therapy in treating PTSD.
CBD taken sublingually or orally in doses of 5 mg to 10 mg twice daily is a common daytime approach for coping with PTSD. Combinations of CBD with low-dose THC also seems to show promise. When doing so, look for a CBD:THC ratio of 10:1 or higher. And avoid taking too much CBD in the evening as it can be wake-promoting.

Vaping or smoking are the most common ways of ingesting cannabinoids for PTSD sufferers. Start with low, match-stick size doses of 2.5 mg to 5 mg when doing so until you can establish the lowest effective dose.

Avoid cannabis cultivars high in Pinene as this terpene could be anxiety and memory provoking. Look for varieties containing Linalool and Limonene instead.

23. Restless Leg Syndrome:

Restless leg syndrome is a nervous disorder that causes the incontrollable urge to move one's legs in order to alleviate any pain or discomfort. It can cause a sensation of creeping and crawling in the feet, calves and thighs.

Because CBD is a known to relieve anxiety, low to moderate doses have shown to provide some symptom relief. When taken sublingually or orally at doses of 5 mg to 10 mg, this dosage seems to do the trick. Look for CBD-rich cultivars that have a CBD:THC ratio of 10:1 or higher.

When vaping or smoking CBD products, use 2.5 mg to 7.5 mg per dose several times a day, but avoid evening use if you're sensitive to the wake-inducing effect that CBD can produce in some users.

CBD-rich varieties that contain high levels of the terpenes Myrcene and Caryophyllene should be sought out.

24. Seizure Disorders:

A seizure occurs when abnormal electrical activity in the brain causes an involuntary change in body movement, sensation and behavior. Currently, anti-epilepsy drugs are the main treatment option for seizure disorders like Dravet Syndrome or Epilepsy.

What's exciting about CBD is that it provides a number of anticonvulsant effects with few adverse side reactions. A typical CBD dosage protocol starts with 10 mg doses taken orally several times a day. This is gradually increased until an effective therapeutic dose is reached.

Doses up to 20 mg per kilogram of body weight for children are well tolerated, but this level of dosage needs to be reached gradually over a period of weeks.

CBD-rich varieties like AC/DC, Ringo's Gift and Sour Tsunami are popular amongst adults with seizure disorders. Look for cultivars high in Linalool, which has anticonvulsant effects.

25. Stress:

Stress is the bodies way of reacting to a condition such as a threat, whether real or perceived, a physical challenge or an emotional strain. It manifests itself in the body as a massive release of hormones and chemicals such as adrenalin, cortisol and norepinephrine. Left unchecked it can lead to chronic anxiety or depression.

Next to pain relief, stress is listed amongst the top reasons why both medical and recreational cannabis users take cannabis.

Both CBD and THC can help reduce the effects of stress. Very low doses of THC (around 2 mg) have shown to reduce the symptoms of stress. However, CBD offers benefits that THC alone doesn't offer. For one, CBD is more effective for anxiety-related stress. It also has no psychoactive side effects, which is important for some cannabis users.

Inhaling small doses of cannabis after work or before bedtime is currently the most common approach for managing periodic bouts of stress. A single inhalation is often adequate enough to trigger a calming effect. Should you be using a high-ratio CBD to THC varietal (greater than 10:1), avoid taking too much of this CBD-rich cannabis just prior to bedtime as it may have a wake-promoting effect.

Sublingual doses of cannabis also provide rapid assimilation and stress relief. One option is to look for CBD:THC ratios in the range of 2:1 having 2.5 mg to 5 mg of CBD along with a low dose of 2 mg of THC. Yet another option often used by chronic stress patients is to take 5 mg of CBD twice daily.

CBD varieties containing the terpenes Myrcene, Linalool and Limonene help to increase the overall effectiveness of the medicine.

As you may have noted, some diseases or disorders that could be treated with CBD-rich plants have been left out of the mix, as not enough anecdotal or scientific research has been done to support the use of cannabidiol. So far, so good?

Diseases like Huntington's, Parkinson's, Multiple Sclerosis do benefit from the use of THC-rich cannabis varietals, especially as it relates to pain relief. This may be something of interest for you to explore at a future date as you learn more about the benefits and disadvantages of using certain cannabinoids.

We initially looked at how cannabis could be processed to create a variety of products that can be inhaled, ingested or applied to the skin. We then touched on a 4-step process of selecting good quality buds. Following this, you were introduced to ten CBD-rich cannabis varieties to consider for your personal use. And finally, we looked at those ailments that cannabis has helped better control and manage as part of an overall health plan. I don't know about you, but I'm dancing around Gangnam Style - excited about the prospect of there being some concrete solutions to what ails us. Now it's time to see how we can identify a consistent quality supply of medicinal cannabis.

How do I select a medical marijuana dispensary?

Medical marijuana products can be either purchased locally from a reputable dispensary or purchased online. Let's first take a look at how to find a dispensary that'll provide you with a consistent supply of top-quality medicine. Then, we'll delve into the pros and cons of purchasing products online.

Whether you're planning on going to a licensed dispensary or one that is not governed by any legislation, the process of doing your due diligence before buying any products is the same. To help you narrow down your choices and find a reputable, reliable dispensary, here are six selection criteria to take into consideration.

Criteria #1 Safe and Inviting Storefront.

Does the dispensary have an established presence in the community? Look for those businesses that have been set up in safe neighborhoods and have an "inviting" appearance.

Has the owner invested capital in providing a safe buying experience, pleasurable atmosphere and extensive list of cannabis products and paraphernalia? When you can see that the owner has invested capital in ensuring that the public is in a safe and pleasant shopping environment, this makes the selection process easier for you.

Theft is a concern for many dispensary shop owners. Security guards have become the norm for many establishments.

Criteria #2: Third Party Certification.

Find out whether or not the products being sold have been tested and certified contaminant free. The dispensary's cultivating and processing partners should have PFC certification in the United States (or Health Canada Certification in Canada). In the Excited States, the American Herbal Products Association and the American Herbal Pharmacopeia have quality standards to abide by.

The cannabis being sold should state what the cannabinoid levels are and list any pesticides or herbicides used in the growing process. If you're looking for pure unadulterated cannabis, choose organically grown cannabis where possible. Look for transparency by the dispensary in disclosing as much product information as possible for you to make informed decisions about each product being sold. Makes sense, right?

Criteria #3: Knowledgeable Staff.

How much health care training has the staff had? Unfortunately, according to a study done in 2016 by Stanford University, only about 20% of the U.S. dispensary staff employees have had any sort of medical or health care training suitable for working in the cannabis industry. You may end up knowing more about cannabis than most industry workers after reading this book. Not very reassuring for the industry, but you should be rubbing your pincers together with all the hope of a newborn fly at a Chinese buffet.

Be cautious about product recommendations that seem to fly in the face of logic. Some products could actually exasperate your medical condition. Be proactive by reading as much as you can about what cannabis can and cannot do for you. This book is a first step to becoming enlightened.

Criteria #4: Variety of Selection.

Those dispensaries that have an array of cannabis products to sell do well. Not everyone visiting a "pot shop" is going to buy dried bud to be smoked or vaped. And the fastest growing trend for CBD users is edibles. Whether you're eating a cookie or ingesting a few drops of tincture or oil, many cannabis users are moving away from inhalable products to ingested ones.

Ingesting cannabis can be more discrete and provide the user with longer-lasting effects. This makes edibles a great choice for those individuals who would like to self-medicate during the work day.

Look for shops that cater to this growing segment of the population, especially if you're more inclined to ingest your medicine as opposed to inhaling it during the day.

Criteria #5: Competitive Pricing.

Pricing models for accessing cannabis products can vary significantly depending on the jurisdiction you're residing in. Given the choice, shop around your neighborhood for those dispensaries that offer consistent, competitive pricing for their products.

Does the shop seem to have a steady flow of clientele that'll keep prices in check? Healthy businesses are those with a loyal customer base. With increasing sales and consistent revenues, many owners are able to pass on the savings to their clientele base. Not unlike a company like Costco being able to keep their margins thin because of the volume of shoppers coming in through their front doors.

The marijuana market is becoming a commodity-based, international industry. Production and processing costs are on the decline. This means that over time, the cost of purchasing your favorite products should drop. I haven't been this happy with this prospect since I learned how to use the toilet myself.

Criteria #6: Membership Agreement.

In some jurisdictions, cannabis can only be sold to individuals holding a valid marijuana license. If you are living in such a jurisdiction, does the dispensary have a membership agreement?

The agreement should spell out things like:
1. Providing a valid marijuana license with any purchase.
2. Agreeing not to give or sell any purchases to other individuals.
3. Where you can obtain further product information.
4. How to lodge a complaint.

Following these six selection criteria should give you greater confidence in buying cannabis products locally.

Should I purchase marijuana online?

Online shopping is a growing trend world-wide and the cannabis industry is tapping into this lucrative way of doing business. No longer do cannabis businesses need to pay the added expense of having brick and mortar shops set up around the country when it can all be done from one central facility.

The challenge is finding a reputable company that is going to provide you with what you desire. According to a 2017 University of Pennsylvania study looking into just this issue, almost 26% of supposed CBD-rich products sold online contained lower doses than indicated on the packaging. Bottom line? You may not be getting any therapeutic effect with too low a concentration of CBD.

Unfortunately, these inconsistencies will continue in the industry due to a lack of regulation by the U.S. Food and Drug Administration. Testing any products purchased online yourself can become cost prohibitive. Should you decide to take this route, look for laboratories that have passed the ISO 17025 certification process. Just like online dispensaries, testing facilities can vary widely in their evaluations.

If you're going to order product online, your best bet is to verify what sort of web presence and reputation the online dispensary has. Does the website look like it was professionally done or set up by a 10-year old? Has the website been up for a significant period of time? Does it educate viewers on cannabis products and current best practices? Are there any purchase guarantees or return policies? Currently, the onus is on you to do some preliminary investigation before buying online.

If you're living in Canada, any government-operated online dispensary will have products that have been tested, approved for sale, and labeled accordingly. The legalization of cannabis on a federal level in Canada has forced cultivators and producers to comply with strict production guidelines set up by Health Canada.

Why holistic health care may be the answer?

I've eluded to the importance of using a multi-faceted approach to better manage whatever ailment you're currently having to contend with. Holistic health care is an integrated approach that incorporates wellness strategies that treat the whole body, not just the symptoms of what ails you.

As I've mentioned already, cannabis is not a "cure" for disease. However, when it's integrated into a total health care approach for treating disease, the probability of success increases dramatically.

And what does an all-encompassing approach to health care look like? Glad you asked.

A simple breakdown of the areas where by you could improve the quality of your life are:
1. Physical Fitness.
2. Healthy Diet and Nutrition.
3. Relaxation and Rest.
4. Elimination of Toxins.

1. Physical Fitness:

We've become a sedentary society over the past 30 years. Unfortunately for most people, physical activity is low on their priority list as something that they should be doing. However, the body requires a certain amount of physical activity in order to remain strong and resistant against disease and illness.

If you're currently not getting in a 45-minute walk, hike, bike, cross country ski, snowshoe, paddle, or integrated gym workout 4 times a week, you're doing your body a disservice. Over time your body's ability to perform simple tasks like walking up a flight of stairs, playing outdoors with the kids, or carrying your groceries out to your car become a real physical challenge. Can you relate to this?

It's never too late to improve your fitness level. In fact, many illnesses improve over time when physical activity is integrated into one's overall health plan. For example, fibromyalgia and arthritis patients often experience less pain and discomfort when regular aerobic exercise is a part of their lifestyle. A case in point is my wife, who needs fewer pain killers during the day when daily exercise is a part of her routine.

2. Healthy Diet and Nutrition:

We live in a society of convenience, which shows up more so in the food industry than anywhere else. People have busy lives with both spouses often having to work in order to make ends meet. It's definitely easier and more convenient to pick up a pre-packaged meal when you're strapped for time. Unfortunately, it has been the demise of far too many in society.

Maybe the old adage "what you eat is what you are" has some truth. Nearly 60% of the population is either overweight or obese. Highly-processed foods and poor eating habits are the main culprits. It's true that processed food tastes really good. Who would buy a product that didn't taste scrumptious? These products are designed to be that way with high levels of fat, sugar and salt. And they're inexpensive to purchase, to boot.

There is a better alternative. Consider making more of a concerted effort to eat whole foods on a daily basis, with most of your diet being vegetable based. Focus on picking up food items that have experienced little or no processing. And you need not go full-tilt boogie into thinking you "have to" do this every day. Old habits are hard to change. Even if you're only successful a few times a week, it's a start.

You'll be amazed how you'll feel after a few weeks of eating healthier. For years now, we've been making a green drink smoothie made up primarily of spinach, cucumber, avocado, mint, apple and berries. Not only is this concoction delicious, it's also nutritious.

3. Relaxation and Sleep:

In our busy worlds of living in a concrete jungle, we often don't take the time to enjoy the finer points of life. We're stressed out beyond belief trying to make ends meet, to cope with increasing physical demands or to deal with emotional challenges. We rarely take the time to stop and literally smell the roses.

We're losing our ability to clear the mind and relax, which eventually affects our sleep and how restful we feel in the morning. The simple act of taking a short walk in the company of Mother Nature does wonders for the psyche, as do daily activities like meditation, visualization and yoga.

Getting adequate and proper sleep is a challenge for many. Too often we're plugged into our electronic devises into the wee hours of the morning. It's no wonder we feel so crappy in the morning as if a steamroller ran over our bodies during the night.

Proper sleep hygiene requires that we change our current sleep habits to be more conducive to getting a good sleep. Begin winding down your body an hour or so before you would like to fall asleep. Start by turning down the lights, shutting off all bright electronic devices, and having things set up for your morning routine. Now your body is able to better transition from a wakeful state to a sleep-inducing one.

Rather than watch TV or be on your computer, consider reading a magazine or book until you begin to feel sleepy. Should noise be a factor, look at using a white noise device in the bedroom. And should lights keep you up at night, blackout curtains may do the trick.

As previously mentioned, small doses of cannabis consumed prior to bedtime may also help induce sleep, allowing your body and mind to decompress and relax.

4. Elimination of Toxins:

Toxins come in all forms - the food we eat, the water we drink, the air we breathe, the chemicals we touch. It's the long-term exposure to low doses of toxins that's associated with many types of disease, especially cancers.

When you make a concerted effort to identify and avoid contact with known toxins in your living and work environment, you've taken an important step towards creating a holistically healthy you.

One simple step is to avoid products in the grocery store that contain preservatives, stabilizers, colorants and conditioners. If you can't pronounce the ingredient on the label, maybe you shouldn't be consuming it, especially if there are alternative choices.

Choose chemical cleaners based on how toxic they could be to you, your loved ones and the environment. Is there a healthier alternative that might be effective? It's the repeated exposure to many of these over-the-counter chemical products that plays havoc on our immune systems.

The bottom line is that by reducing many of the risk factors addressed in the above section, you can arrest and even reverse the effects of disease and illness in your life. A holistic approach to health and wellness is always the best course of action. And you need not make drastic changes to see positive results. Start by selecting one area in each of the four covered that you could subtly change today. Those small steps taken today eventually translate into massive health gains down the road.

With this in mind, let's take a look at how you could use the most popular cannabis products to help you better manage what ails you in conjunction with a holistic health care approach.

Chapter 4: How Should I Use CBD-Rich Products?

Few health care professionals and most novice cannabis users have little idea as to how to dose and administer cannabis. The key factor to using any cannabis product comes down to determining the "lowest effective" dose that'll provide you with relief or your desired effect.

As you may have already surmised, dose guidance depends on both the method of ingestion and the potency of the product.

I should point out that THC taken in high doses can lead to intoxication, whereas CBD is easier on the body at higher doses since it produces no psychoactive effect. This is why recreational users of THC-rich marijuana are cautioned to go easy on dosing, especially when using concentrates like hash, wax, and shatter.

On the other hand, CBD concentrates pose less of a dosing problem. This is one reason why the real growth in the cannabis industry is coming in the form of CBD concentrates that can be added to a variety of products such as edibles, creams, beverages, oils and tinctures.

In the next section that covers how to discretely grow your own medicine, you'll also learn how to create many of the above-mentioned products. Growing your own quality medicine not only saves you money that would otherwise be spent on retail products, but it's fun watching your "kids" grow from tiny seedlings to bushy, resinous adults. I don't know about you, but this makes me happier than the monks who discovered the word was "celebrate" not "celibate".

Dosing is individual dependent. Your least effective dose is best determined through trial and error with accurate documentation as to the amounts and effects of each dosage. Your ability to come up with your particular effective dose is going to be based on your experience with cannabis, how healthy you are as an individual, and your genetics.

If you're a first-time user who has not been exposed to any cannabinoids before, your endo-cannabinoid system may not yet be primed to benefit from ingesting cannabinoids. I know that my first-time using cannabis did nothing for me. It wasn't until I repeated the experience a couple of times before I was able to see the benefits manifest themselves. This may be the case for you. Patience is key in this situation. Allow your body to adjust and prime itself for future cannabinoid ingestion.

Dosing calculations simplified:

How much CBD enters your body is based on the following three factors:
1. The quantity of product being used per dosage,
2. The percentage of CBD/THC in the product being used, and
3. How efficient the method of delivery is in actually delivering the cannabinoids and terpenes into the bloodstream.

The last factor is one that is hard to measure with much accuracy. It largely depends on one's ability to ingest the cannabinoids contained in the product at an optimal level.

We do know that some methods of ingestion are more efficient in delivering cannabinoids to the body. Unfortunately, a lack of peer-reviewed research exists that can provide concrete dosing recommendations. More research needs be done that looks into dosing levels for various means of ingesting cannabis for the various ailments that we face.

The recommendations that follow are based on anecdotal reports in the industry as opposed to peer-reviewed scientific studies. Here's a rough guideline that may help you in assessing delivery efficiency:
1. Vaping Dried Bud: 75%+
2. Sublingual Tincture/Oil: 75%+
3. Smoking Concentrates: 50%+
4. Smoking Dried Bud: 25%+
5. Edibles & Beverages: 25%+
6. Topical Applications: 10%+

What this all means is that you'll need more of a product as the body's ability to absorb the cannabinoids decreases in efficiency. For example, you'll require more dried bud when smoking a cannabis cigarette as opposed to vaping dried bud. Start with the base value above and increase it when you're able to optimize cannabinoid delivery with the delivery method selected.

In general, vaping, smoking and sublingual applications provide the fastest means for the body to absorb cannabinoids and terpenes making them easier to titrate dosing. Eating or drinking products containing cannabis is slower and dosing becomes more erratic.

We all process foods at different rates of absorption and efficiency levels in extracting cannabinoids. Your weight, diet, metabolism and health all factor into the equation. With this in mind, let's walk through a couple of dosing examples:

Example #1 - Vaping CBD Bud:
You've purchased an "eighth of weed" (3.5 grams) of ACDC dried bud from your local dispensary. The packaging indicates that the CBD-rich bud has been tested to contain 20% CBD. If 1 gram is the same as 1000 milligrams (mg) and you have 3.5 grams of dried bud, then your package has a maximum total of 700 mg of CBD (3500 mg x 20%).

You decide to grind a very small quantity of dried bud and weigh out 0.05 grams (50 mg) that you place in your vaporizer. This small amount represents $1/70^{th}$ of your total stash, which equates to a maximum dose of 10 mg of CBD ($1/70^{th}$ of 700 mg).

You "guestimate" that your vaporizer and proper vaping technique will deliver a 75% efficiency rate of getting CBD into your bloodstream. This means that you would be able to ingest 7.5 mg of CBD (10 mg x 75%).

As you can surmise from this example a very small amount of cannabis can deliver an effective dose of cannabinoids. And absorption efficiency plays a part in how much product to use. Here's a second example to sink your teeth into.

Example #2 - CBD Oil taken Sublingually:
You have a small bottle of CBD oil that indicates that a serving size of 10 drops of oil provides 20 mg of CBD. The suggested CBD starting dosage that your health care practitioner has suggested you take for your particular condition is between 5 and 10 mg.

You conservatively "guestimate" that taken sublingually, a "serving size" of 10 drops would provide 15 mg of CBD (75% of 20 mg). The 75% represents how efficient this delivery method is in delivering the cannabinoids to your system.

However, your health care professional is recommending a lower dose to start with than 15 mg. How much should you take?

If 10 drops would only provide 15 mg of CBD because of a loss of absorption efficiency, then you would need to take roughly 4 drops to get about 5 mg of CBD in that dose (5 mg/15 mg x 10 drops).

Your ultimate goal is to establish the lowest possible dose that you require for a given delivery method. And this is usually accomplished through trial and error. However, if you're inclined to err on the side of caution, then initially measuring out your dosages as in the above examples may provide greater insights. A digital scale accurate to 0.01 grams can be purchased locally or on Amazon for about $14.

Top 6 cannabis delivery methods:

Let's touch on the most popular methods of delivery of CBD-rich cannabis, what you can expect and how to both efficiently and effectively use each product. Here are the delivery methods that we'll cover:
1. Smoking
2. Vaping
3. Smoking Concentrates
4. Sublingual Ingestion
5. Edibles & Beverages
6. Topical Applications.

First in the lineup is smoking dried cannabis herb.

1. Smoking:

Smoking dried ground-up herb is the most common way cannabis is consumed today since it's easy to use and fast-acting. A small ground-up quantity of dried herb is rolled in cigarette paper and then smoked just like a cigarette.

A hand-held grinder designed to coarsely grind cannabis buds is a worthwhile investment. Chop up your cannabis buds using the grinder so that you avoid using your fingers since cannabinoid-rich resin tends to adhere to them.

These pocket-size devices prep the cannabis so that you can get the most out of each dose. Look for devices made of resistant aircraft aluminum having precision-designed teeth designed for properly shredding your bud.

To get an idea as to what devices are out in the market, visit your local cannabis retailer or pop onto Amazon to check out your options for a cannabis herb grinder. A well-made device should cost you between $10 and $20 US.

Cannabinoids from smoked buds immediately enter the bloodstream, which makes it easy to adjust dosing. Peak blood levels of cannabinoids are reached within five to ten minutes of inhalation. If the first small dose that you take proves to be insufficient, you can always take another one after waiting several minutes for the first dose to take full effect.

The downside of smoking any cannabis is that you're also ingesting harmful chemicals from the burning plant matter, not unlike some of the toxins from tobacco smoke.

When smoking cannabis, inhale slowly and evenly through your mouth filling your lungs until almost full, pause for a split second, then, quickly exhale any cannabis smoke. Avoid deeply inhaling and holding cannabis smoke in the lungs for long periods of time as this technique may prove harmful to your lungs. Focus on a smooth, even draw as you inhale followed by a rapid exhalation.

An alternative to smoking cannabis cigarettes is to use a small cannabis pipe. These discrete "one-hitters" are often made of borosilicate glass. Cleaning them becomes a snap. Adjusting dosing is much easier using a small pipe, rather than smoking a cigarette.

When using a pipe bowl, place a small quantity of ground up dried bud into the bowl, then try to heat the bud gently from the edge. Care should be taken not to ignite the ground bud as a visible flame indicates that both beneficial terpenes and cannabinoids are being burned off.

You can check out various designs at your local cannabis retailer or explore a few options online. A simple glass smoking pipe can be purchased on Amazon for about $15.

Beyond the scope of this book is the use of cannabis pipes that use a water system to cool and filter the smoke. They do provide a more pleasurable experience, but one must factor in both the purchase price, ease of use and discrete use of the pipe into the investment equation.

Pricing of cannabis buds is based on a certain dollar value per gram. For example, you may see Harlequin being sold for $9/gram at your local dispensary. Dried cannabis buds come in various package sizes with the most common sizing's being 1 gram, 3.5 grams (1/8 ounce), 7 grams (1/4 ounce), 10 grams (1/3 ounce), and 14 grams (1/2 ounce). Following me so far?

2. Vaping:

Cannabis cigarettes, which are known as joints or spliffs, are losing popularity amongst medicinal cannabis users. There is often no need to smoke an entire cigarette to get the beneficial effects from our high-potency cannabis today.

Vaping is a better alternative to smoking. These electronic devices can be as small as a pen or as large as a kettle. They can be found in portable, handheld and desktop models. Portable vaporizers are great for vaporizing dried bud. They offer the biggest bang for your buck in being convenient, discreet and versatile. Handheld vape pens can be either refillable or disposable models. They're often best for oil concentrates and wax. Being small and discreet, they're also inexpensive. Desktop versions also exist for those looking for a home device capable of delivering.

When my wife and I vape at home, we typically use about 0.05 grams (50 mg) of dried bud when we vape, which is a lot less than a typical joint. Yes, you do have the upfront cost of investing in a vaporizer. However, since the dried herb is heated just to the point of vaporizing the cannabinoids contained within, fewer harmful or harsh chemicals are inhaled. Also, vaporization of the cannabinoids and terpenes at just the right temperature makes it more efficient than smoking dried bud.

As the price of vaporizers drops, you'll see an increasing demand and use of these devices in the future. As with smoking, vaped cannabinoids quickly enter the bloodstream within several seconds of inhalation.

The devices entering the market today are discrete looking and often fit comfortably and unobtrusively into a coat pocket. All vaporizers have a heating element, a bowl or compartment for holding the cannabis herb or concentrate, and a way of catching and drawing in the vapor. Most models use some sort of a mouthpiece for this.

Vaporizers are designed to rapidly heat the cannabis to a temperature range of 330°F to 375°F (165°C to 190°C) at which point the cannabinoids and terpenes are vaporized for inhalation. This temperature range is well below the 400°F mark that causes the release of tars and toxic compounds. The more expensive vaporizers have a temperature control system that allows you to finely tune your vaping experience to best suit your needs.

When using a vaporizer with dried herb, pack finely ground herb into the bowl. Ensure that there is an even distribution that'll produce a more complete vaporization of the cannabinoids and terpenes. You want to expose as much surface area to heat and air flow.

When using a vaporizer designed for concentrates like wax or oil, these devices often use pre-filled cartridges that can be quickly and easily replaced. This is one reason why inexpensive vape pens are gaining in popularity.

As in smoking cannabis cigarettes, focus on a slow steady draw with a rapid exhale. You may need to draw longer and softer than you would if you were smoking a joint.

When purchasing a vaporizer, you should base your decision on many if not all of these factors:
1. Price point.
2. Ease of use and cleaning.
3. Use with dried bud and/or concentrates.
4. Discreteness.
5. Temperature adjustability.
6. Battery longevity.
7. Durability.
8. Warranty and company reputation.

Let's look at a handful of examples of devices found in the three major categories of vaporizers:
1. Portable Vaporizers.
2. Vaporizer Pens.
3. Desktop Vaporizers.

(a) Portable Vaporizers.

Dry herb vaporizers are the most common and easiest vaping devices to use. These devices can heat your bud by direct contact with the heating element, known as conduction heating, or by passing heated air over your bud by the means of convection. Less expensive devices often use a conduction heating element, which can cause combustion of your bud (burning as opposed to vaporizing). Using a more expensive convection vaporizer avoids this problem. Here are a couple of popular portable vaporizers to explore.

Pax 3:
The Pax 3 is a dual-use vaporizer that can vape both dried bud and wax concentrates. It has four pre-set heat features and being Bluetooth compatible you can customize your settings with your smartphone.

The compact design even allows the mouthpiece to hide within the top of the device. Besides being discreet, the Pax 3 has a quick heating time of about 15 seconds.

The one downside is that being so versatile and adjustable comes with a price. This is definitely an "investment" piece. Suggested retail price: $250 US.

Firefly 2:
The Firefly 2 has a light, compact design and is made of quality material throughout with a titanium alloy heating element and all-glass vapor path. Like the Pax 3, it is a dual-use vaporizer as well.

The biggest advantage is the fast recharge time (45 minutes). Like the Pax 3, it's a programmable unit. It's also a pricey piece of equipment. Suggested retail price: $330 US.

(b) Vaporizer Pens.

Vaporizer pens are small, portable vaping devices often designed to be used with refillable cartridges that contain oil concentrates or even wax. They're typically smaller and more discrete than portable vaporizers. If the vape pen is designed to be used with dried herb, it won't be as powerful nor as efficient as a portable device that's designed to produce a quality vapor. What the vape pen lacks in quality, it makes up in convenience and price. Here are two to check out.

Mig Vapor's Herb-E:
Despite being one of the smallest dry-herb vape pens on the market, the Herb-E packs a punch. The pen features two modes of operation, a yellow mode for good flavor production and a red mode for producing a denser vapor. It has a durable, carbon-fibre exterior and easy-to-operate, one-button control. This device can also vape concentrates, when a chamber for concentrates is ordered separately.

The downside? It does have a low vapor production, which may not be adequate for some users. The Herb-E also has limited settings with only two pre-sets available, unlike most portable vaporizers. Suggested retail price: $60 US.

Mig Vapor's WASP:
The WASP is one of the best concentrate, vape pens currently available. It works best with waxes of medium consistency, but can be used with oils, shatters and "budder". (More on these concentrates in a moment).

The WASP is built to last, being made of high-quality carborundum and stainless-steel components. It has a consistent power output that heats the coils in a matter of seconds with a simple, one-button activation. Unfortunately, it doesn't have any adjustable settings. Suggested retail price: $60 US.

(c) Desktop Vaporizers.

Table-top or desktop vaporizers are larger, more powerful devices. They're also more expensive as compared to portable devices. You can't carry these devices around discreetly like a pen or handheld device. However, they do offer better performance, rich flavor and fast recharge times.

Storz & Bickel's Volcano Classic:
The Volcano is the most widely used vaporizer in dispensaries, hospitals and compassion clubs. And it looks like a volcano to boot. It's a forced-air, plug-in, desktop unit that can vaporize dried bud, oils and waxes. The unit has precise convection heating, ensuring that no combustion takes place. It also has precise temperature settings and control.

Once the device has heated up, turning on a second switch turns on the air pump, which forces filtered, heated air through the herb chamber and into a collection bag. By disconnecting the bag from the Volcano, the user can press their lips against the bag's mouthpiece and gently inhale releasing the vapor. The unit comes with five easy-to-use balloon bags that are filled with vapor and inhaled during operation. Each bag has a life expectancy of 50 to 100 fills.

Besides an initial learning curve for using the Volcano, the biggest deterrent may be the sticker price. Suggested retail price: $479 US.

Storz & Bickel's Plenty:
The Plenty is a smaller "hand-held" version of the Volcano that comes with a 12-foot, 3-prong electrical cord. It too can use dried herb or wax concentrates. This German-made, medical-grade, quality unit has adjustable temperature settings. It has a wide, shallow, filling chamber that produces potent vapor quickly. The vapor is drawn up through a metal coil that cools the vapor before it reaches the mouthpiece.

As with the Volcano, both the high price and high maintenance, factor into your buying decision. Also, you may need to attach an extension cord should you be using the device in a group setting where its likely you'll be passing the device around. Suggested retail price: $249 US.

These examples of popular devices should provide you with a brief introduction to the world of vaping should you decide to head down that path at a future time. Moving on to …

3. Smoking Concentrates:

You may have seen small groups of cannabis users gathered around strange glass contraptions that bubble clouds of white vapor through them with each hit. A growing trend among recreational marijuana users is to smoke concentrates in minute quantities or "dabs", hence the term dabbing. These concentrates being devoid of organic matter are less harmful than ingesting bud alone, which can harbor bacteria, mold and fungi.

However, being in a concentrated form, they're harder to titrate dosing since the potent cannabinoid levels are much higher than in dried bud. Another downside is that smoking concentrates does require some special tools that may or may not appeal to you.

The simplest set-up is a "one-hitter" glass cannabis pipe that has been fitted with a ceramic insert designed to hold the concentrate. One step up from this is a dabbing rig. At a minimum, you'll need two basic special tools a dabbing tool, "wand" or "nail" and a special (water) pipe that has been modified to consume concentrates.

The dabber is used to titrate a small dosage of concentrate that will then be heated to the point of vaporization. The hot vapor is then typically drawn through a glass water pipe to be cooled before inhaling.

Heating can be either externally using a small butane torch or internally as part of the glass dabbing rig that has been fitted with a shallow bowl that's heated electrically.

Dabbers are made of inert substances like quartz, titanium or ceramic since they can withstand high heat without giving off any toxic fumes themselves. When using a nail or a dabber, a small quantity of concentrate is placed on the tip to be heated by a butane torch. These are the same type of butane torches that are often used to light cigars. You want to avoid using a cheap Bic lighter as it tends to make smoked concentrates taste terrible.

Concentrates can be made a number of ways. They can have a glass or wax-like consistency, hence the terms shatter, "budder" and crumble.

The most common industrial process that produces the safest concentrates uses pressurized, liquified CO_2 gas, which is easily removed from the resulting concentrate.

Besides CO_2 extraction, another solvent, butane can be used to produce shatter, wax and budder.

And, the latest technology uses a hyperbaric chamber with pressurized nitrogen to produce more flavorful, aromatic concentrates. Hyperbaric chambers are used to treat divers suffering from the bends.

Dabbing results in a rapid, intense effect in the body. It can be extremely disorienting or overwhelming for some individuals who take too big of a hit. It's easy to over medicate when dabbing, so dose control is essential. However, with both smoking and vaping cannabis, the long-term effects and benefits tend to wear off faster than with other methods of ingestion.

Concentrates are often packaged in small silicon jars that come in 3 mL, 5 mL and 7 mL sizes. Silicon is often used as opposed to glass or metal as concentrates stick less to the surface making these storage containers more user friendly.

Should you like to explore this fascinating area of cannabis use, take a look at what's available online. Amazon has glass water pipe's for as low as $30.

4. Sublingual Ingestion:

Another common approach to taking medicinal cannabis is sublingually (placing cannabinoids just under the tongue) using an oil, tincture or spray. Sublingual cannabis products typically come in more potent forms, where a small dose goes a long way and ingestion of the cannabinoids occurs quickly, usually within minutes. It may not be as fast as vaping, but it does have the distinct advantage of not irritating the respiratory system like smoking can.

Cannabis oil gained notoriety when Rick Simpson promoted his "Phoenix Tears" as a cure for cancer back in the 90's. It's often prepared at home by soaking cannabis bud in a solvent like ethyl alcohol, separating the cannabinoid-rich filtrate from any solid organic matter and gently boiling the solvent away leaving a cannabinoid-rich viscous oil that can be administered under the tongue.

Tinctures can be made by dissolving bud in alcohol or glycerin, filtering off any solids and using the resulting solution. A few drops of concentrated solution placed under the tongue and allowed to slowly absorb into the bloodstream is the common approach to administration.

You'll often feel the effects coming on within 5 minutes of ingestion, making it relatively easy to adjust dosing. Full effects should be felt within 20 minutes. Once you've used a particular product a few times, it'll be easy to determine the right dose. A well-made tincture or oil is an enjoyable, easy and effective way to take cannabinoids without smoking.

The most common type of tincture uses alcohol as the solvent, which has the added advantage of being a good preservative. Glycerine is also becoming more common as a tincture base, especially for those individuals sensitive to the alcohol base.

When buying tinctures, look for amber or cobalt blue glass bottles, sometimes called "Boston rounds". Avoid plastic bottles as the solvent will eventually react with the plastic. Cannabis tinctures are often sold in droplet bottle sizes of 10 mL, 15 mL, and 30 mL.

All oils and tinctures should be kept at a minimum in a cool, dark place for storage. Ideally, a refrigerator will slow down the cannabinoid degradation the best.

Commercial spray applicators containing a propellent and CBD-rich liquid concentrate can also be purchased for buccal ingestion.

5. Edibles & Beverages:

Eating food products containing cannabis is a tasty effective way of taking your medicine. Eating cannabis products is more discrete than vaping or smoking since there are no signs of smoke or vapor being produced. The biggest advantage is that oral ingestion produces a longer-lasting effect than vaping or smoking. You can expect edibles to last about twice as long as vaped or smoked cannabis.

However, determining the optimal dose can be tricky. We all have different rates of metabolism. As a simple rule of thumb, edibles ingested on an empty stomach often enter the bloodstream within 15 to 25 minutes, reaching peak levels within 30 to 90 minutes and lasting for up to 6 or 7 hours. The effects do last longer and fade more slowly than other forms of ingestion.

Another challenge with dosing is that since we process foods at different metabolic rates of efficiency, there may be a tendency to ingest too much product thinking that the first dose was inadequate when in fact it was taking a bit longer to enter the bloodstream.

Getting the right dose is more important with edibles than vaped or smoked products. The amount of food you eat, how it was prepared and the concentration level of cannabinoids factor into how you'll react. This is why it's important to know how much you're ingesting before starting.

With cannabis being an herb, it can be added directly to soups and stews at the tail-end of the cooking process. Excessive heating of cannabis in the cooking process destroys the cannabinoids and terpenes. Also, cooking with dried bud, kief or hash can produce strong odors especially at higher temperatures. Having a carbon air filter handy, helps. Using ginger, cloves, cinnamon, nutmeg, orange extract or chocolate in a recipe helps to mask any odors, as well as kick up the flavor a notch.

Both kief (dried resinous glands containing cannabinoids) and hash (pressed kief) can be sprinkled on dishes as a condiment. Just ensure that you blend the kief or hash consistently and evenly into the dish so as to avoid any "over-seasoned" spots. They can also be added to various oils and butter to be used in salad dressings or for heating foods at low temperatures.

Cannabis capsules can also be purchased or made. Known as canna-caps, they are usually size "0" gelatin capsules filled with a cannabis concentrate (like kief or hash) that has been dissolved in an oil-based medium like coconut or olive oil. Coconut oil has the advantage of being solid at room temperature.

Should you be using kief for making your own capsules, use the smaller size "0" capsules that'll hold a maximum of 0.35 grams (350 mg) of filler as opposed to the larger "00" capsules that'll hold twice as much (750 mg). The smaller size allows for a more precise dosage being administered. This is often my preferred means of taking medication at night when I want to sleep like a baby - curled up in a ball, thumb in my mouth while gently sobbing.

Canna-caps have the distinct advantage of being conveniently packaged and easy to use. You can take them on their own without having to eat any other food. Also, dosing becomes easier than with other food items.

Foods prepared with whole milk or soy products containing the emulsifier lecithin speed the absorption of cannabinoids in the body. So, be cautious when you decide to have that salmon pasta recipe made with a delicious cream and butter sauce.

By far the most popular commercially made food items are cannabis cookies, candies and other treats. Eaten as a snack, they're absorbed faster by the body than a heavy meal. However, just because that chocolate chip cookie tastes great doesn't mean you should over-indulge. Choose modest portions until you know how your body is going to react. Should you have a sweet tooth, ensure that you keep those delectable treats out of the reach of children and pets. Clearly label all of your cannabis food items to avoid accidental ingestion.

As well, please don't serve "spiked" foods to guests without letting them know and possibly providing an alternative dish to sample. It's a good idea when serving any cannabis dessert product to have an alternative on hand so no one goes overboard. The worst-case scenario is that your guests will all fall asleep with smiles on their faces from over-eating.

The most common packaging sizes for a variety of edibles is in plastic containers of 4, 8, 12, 16 and 24 ounces. Keep any edibles in sealed, opaque containers that can be stored in the refrigerator or freezer. You'll want to protect these cannabinated foods from exposure to oxygen and light.

The beverage industry is in its infancy when it comes to incorporating cannabis concentrates into various types of beverages. Beverages infused with CBD-rich extracts from non-alcoholic energy drinks and herbal teas to robust red wines and hoppy beers are making their appearance.

We're seeing more and more CBD-rich beverages entering the global market. Since CBD is non-psychoactive and does not interact with alcohol like THC, it has become the choice of many beverage companies.

It's interesting to note that where recreational cannabis has become legal, beer sales have fallen 10 to 15% in those jurisdictions. This can be expected as both industries share a similar demographic profile. Hence, the movement underfoot by some of the major alcoholic beverage producers to look at introducing cannabis-infused beers, wines and spirits. Doing so opens up another, previously unheard-of market to consumers. Do I hear a little voice in my head saying, "investment opportunity"?

Strong-flavored products work best to mask any vegetative cannabis taste. And many of these alcoholic beverages are best aged before bottling to ensure that the maximum amount of CBD will be extracted. Aging also mellows out the cannabis flavour in beverages like wine and beer.

When consuming these products, do so cautiously as you would any edible. The relatively slow digestion time may have you thinking that having a 3rd bottle of CBD-infused beer is okay, only to be "couch-locked" an hour later. Mamma Mia!

6. Topical Applications:

CBD applied to the skin in the form of a topical cream, lotion or oil can provide localized relief for certain skin conditions and for joint inflammation. Even migraines have been treated with some success with the application of salves to the temples, neck and forehead.

Since cannabinoids are readily dissolved in oils, alcohol and glycerin, most topical products will use a combination of these three carriers in their formulation. Go easy on the first application should you be using a topical application for the first time. Some individuals will develop an allergic reaction to certain ingredients found within the topical formulation.

As well, look for topical products that contain a significant amount of CBD in order to provide the relief that you're seeking. Topical preparations are not as efficient a delivery method of cannabinoids as vaping, smoking or ingesting, so you'll want a formulation that has a higher concentration of active ingredients.

If you are in a profession that requires drug testing, topicals may be a good choice since they do not produce the same cannabis metabolites that can be detected with current drug tests. Besides, most drug tests focus on THC levels (the psychoactive cannabinoid) as opposed to CBD.

Opening up the skin's pores with heat such as a hot bath, a shower, or a heating pad helps with absorption. And gentle massage of the area affected creates friction which helps to transport the CBD-rich salve or oil into joints. Covering the area can also increase absorption. Trans-dermal patches are entering the market with this property in mind. Also, topicals containing alcohol may be absorbed better as the alcohol opens up the skin's pores.

Pure, concentrated cannabis oil like Rick Simpson oil, used as a topical treatment for certain types of skin cancer has been shown to reduce tumours. The cannabinoids seem to selectively cut off the blood flow to the tumor, causing the cancerous cells to die off naturally while limiting the spread of other cells. Massaging cannabis oil into the affected area and then covering it is the preferred method of application.

Avoid products containing parabens and petroleum-based chemicals that can cause other health problems.

The most common sizes of wide-mouthed, glass ointment jars used for topical CBD formulations is 0.5, 1, 2 and 8-ounce containers.

Top take-aways:

In this section of the book, you've learned about the important interplay between cannabinoids and terpenes in healing the body. You've picked up a myriad of tips on how to buy CBD-rich products, which varieties of cannabis to possibly try and what ailments may be effectively treated with CBD. We've also touched on six cost-effective delivery methods to consider that'll provide you with the optimal relief that you're seeking for what ails you.

In this next section, I'll take you by the hand and walk you through how to set up a discrete closet grow that'll produce your own quality medicine. You'll learn about what you need and don't need, along with what you should do and should avoid in order to grow successful crop after successful crop. Finally, you'll learn how to produce some of the products we've already discussed using your own cannabis. Not only will you be able to save a pretty penny growing your own medicine, but you'll also have control over its purity and future use. Hang onto your wigs and toupees because this next section is so powerful, it'll blow them right off your head. There's nothing like saving thousands of dollars each year producing your own quality medicine.

Section 3: How to Stealthily Grow Cannabis Indoors.

The focus of this section of your book is to provide you with a step-by-step guide as to how to create a discrete, "closet" grow.
You'll learn about:
1. What are the benefits of growing your own medicine?
2. Why an indoor closet grow and what do you need?
3. How much can you expect to spend on equipment?
4. How do you create an optimal grow environment indoors?
5. What do you need to do to produce a variety of medicinal products?

By the end of this section, you'll be able to grow and process your own medicine within the confines of a small space. Once you get into the routine of periodically producing your own medicine, what you've initially invested in setting up your equipment will be recouped quickly from the cost savings of having to buy these CBD-rich products in the market.

The first order of business is to explore how you could conceivably set up a discreet grow, what equipment and supplies to buy, and how to set everything up.

Chapter 5: How "Should" I Set Up a Discrete Closet Grow?

Cannabis is a fast-growing "weed" that'll grow under many environmental conditions. In a typical one-light closet grow, you should be able to produce a healthy crop of medicine every 4 months when starting from seed using a typical CBD-rich cannabis strain.

In a nutshell, cannabis likes to be in a temperate climate. And coincidentally, so do most people of the world. Imagine being a cannabis plant overlooking the countryside, growing profusely when the air temperature is around 78°F, the relative humidity hovers just above 50%, there's a light breeze hitting your backside and you're basking in more than of 12 hours of sunlight. Sounds like an enticing cruise vacation.

—

By maintaining these favorable growing conditions, your plant is content to continue producing vegetative growth and could conceivably do so for years. However, this scenario doesn't produce the medicine that we seek.

As with all plants, cannabis thrives when certain growing conditions are met. And since we'll be growing the plant in the confines of a small space, we need to address 4 key factors:

1. Quality and duration of the light source being used.
2. Temperature of the grow space throughout the growing cycle.
3. Amount of humidity during the different phases of plant growth.
4. Air ventilation, circulation and purification.

By manipulating our 4 environmental factors over the growing cycle, we can trick the plant into thinking that its life is about to end. When the temperature, humidity, and light levels decrease both the male and female plants start to produce flowers. The male plant hopes to spread its pollen throughout the female plants so that seeds can be produced, thus continuing the plant's life cycle. Needless-to-say that we need to cull any male plants from our harem of females in our closet grow.

Our goal is to produce the CBD-rich flowers (aka buds) found in the unfertilized female plant. Once the females become fertilized with male pollen, the lack-luster buds being produced are full of seeds. This is not conducive to producing buds with high levels of CBD.

Why grow your own medicine?

Before we delve into how you could conceivably grow your own medicine, let me ask you this: Why would anyone consider growing their own medicine if it's becoming more readily available?

And that's just the point - "having" effective medicine available to you when you need it. Wouldn't you agree? Not everyone reading this how to guide is living in an area where easy and affordable access to quality medicine is just a 10-minute drive away. Hence, the reason why it's important to address this aspect when one is doing some research into how to use CDB.

There are 4 major benefits associated with producing your CBD-rich cannabis plants.

They can be loosely grouped under:

1. Quality control.
2. Cost savings.
3. Gardening green thumb.
4. Sharing the benefits.

Benefit #1: One of the key advantages of growing your own cannabis plants is that you get to control the quality of the medicine you're producing.

You get to regulate all of the nutrients and chemicals that go into a normal grow op. This means choosing between all organic nutrient sources to a using a blend of organic and "synthetic" products known to enhance plant growth and bud development. It means being able to decide on using purified water like reverse osmosis water or just tap water for your grow.

The bud that you'll be producing will be 100% under your control. You'll know what you're getting from each bud. No second guessing as to what pesticides, herbicides, or chemicals may or may not have been used.

True many jurisdictions have strict guidelines as to packaging and labeling cannabis products sold in the retail market where growers are required to list all of the pesticides and herbicides used in the grow.

However, if you live in a jurisdiction that doesn't allow the sale of recreational marijuana, you may find it difficult if near impossible to get this information. Growing your own medicine in a controlled environment provides a solution.

Benefit #2: A huge advantage of growing your own medicine, is that when done properly, you can save a lot of money down the road. Sure, there's the initial cost of investing in your grow op. But you'll be surprised at how inexpensive the entry costs can be in producing quality cannabis at home.

When you take into consideration your initial set up costs, the purchase of seeds or clones, your electrical energy consumption bills, and the bottles of nutrients you'll need, you'll still be able to produce your own cheaper than what you would spend in the retail market.

Until the retail price of a gram of marijuana decreases over time to a point where it sells for less than $5/ gram retail, growing your own has a cost-saving benefit. We're a long way away from having massive producers driving the price of cannabis down from current levels of $10 - $12/ gram so that it becomes an affordable commodity like barley or wheat - both of which can make a fine beer.

Benefit #3: Now, should you be a gardener like the Jolly Green Giant, then your green thumb may serve you well in a cannabis grow.

Some of you may be drawn towards the notion of producing something from Mother Earth that you can be proud of. Gardening can be therapeutic for many and cultivating your own medicine can be even more enticing.

If you like the challenge of nurturing a small seed into something of value down the road that helps you live a healthier life, then by all means consider growing your own cannabis. There's nothing like the feeling of harvesting your first crop of medicine knowing that you or a loved one will be directly benefiting from 4 months of passionate attention. I always get excited like a hamster on a wheel around harvest time. It's rewarding seeing how a handful of seeds can turn into a pound or two of medicine.

Benefit #4: Passion also comes in another form, that of the desire to help others with their struggles. Being a care giver or having a drive to share your talents with those in need can easily be fulfilled by growing your own cannabis with the sole intent of sharing it with loved ones.

How do you add value to society and the world we live in? In all likelihood, it isn't through cannabis. But what if it were? How many of those in need would be grateful of what you've done for them?

You get to share the benefits of cannabis with others, while potentially benefitting from the medicine yourself.

There may be other noble reasons as to why you would want to grow your own medicine. If you feel that this option is a good fit for you after reading the following section, then all the more power to you.

Let's take a look at some ways in which cannabis can be grown and what you need to consider when choosing one particular approach over another.

Why an indoor closet grow?

Let's back up a bit before tackling this puppy. Typically, cannabis is grown commercially in three types of growing environments:

1.   Outdoors.
2.   Greenhouses.
3.   Indoors.

An outdoor grow has the advantage of producing large volumes of marijuana plants under natural environmental conditions at the lowest cost to the producer. Unfortunately, it exposes the crops to pests and easy theft, unless extensive security measures are in place, like crocodiles, land mines and barbed wire.

Greenhouses afford more control over the growing environment, while using natural sunlight to foster plant growth. They also afford more protection against inclement weather and would-be thieves.

An indoor grow captures the entire growing operation within the confines of a building. Buildings tend to be the most secure growing environment. Light, humidity, water, nutrition and even the growing medium are all controlled. This ability to monitor and control plant growing conditions allows for greater consistency in quality production. As with a greenhouse grow, the downside is the initial cost outlay to set up each grow operation since all of the environmental factors have to be addressed.

What should your primary goal be, if you're looking at producing your own home-grown medicine? Good question, R.J.

Your focus should be to establish a discreet indoor closet grow in a <u>simple, easy-to-control environment</u> that <u>produces quality medicine inexpensively</u>.

An indoor closet grow provides you with the following key advantages, over other means:

1. Stealth: The fact that your entire grow operation can be hidden out of sight is a huge advantage should you be in an apartment building, condo unit or basement suite. Landlords, caretakers, friends and even grandpa and grandma will be hard-pressed to know something is aloof. Should you decide to grow your own medicine in a jurisdiction that forbids it, stealth becomes your #1 friend.

2. Small Footprint: You'll be amazed at how much quality, home-grown bud you can produce in the space of a typical 2' x 4' closet. If you're producing what you personally need, you don't require much space. And a spare closet is an easy fit for most.

3. Time Manageable: As you increase the footprint of your grow op, the more challenging it becomes to properly take care of each crop. You'll need to have access to each plant in order to take it from the seedling stage to a flowering plant. It'll also take you longer to feed, water, harvest and process each crop. This is why a 2' x 4' closet grow is the ideal choice for most home growers.

4. Cost Effective: A small footprint grow requires less equipment to purchase up front, thus being a cheaper means of getting into growing. Granted, the larger the grow op the more economical it can potentially become down the road. However, with the modest goal of producing what we expect to use, we'll spend less on our initial investment getting set up. An additional advantage is that a closet grow requires little energy consumption when properly set up. You won't be sending up any red flags by keeping your grow op small.

DIY or pre-fabricated set-up?

You may be tempted to pull a "MacGyver" and consider building your own grow op from a tarp, a roll of duct tape, some scraps of wood and a handful of rusty nails. You may even consider yourself to be a great handyman who has a knack for building something out of nothing.

Resist the urge, Grasshopper. Invest in an indoor grow tent from the start. It'll save you time and frustration down the road when things aren't working out as planned with your tent set-up. Besides, what are you going to do should you have to move things discretely into another apartment or home?

Why invest in a quality grow tent?

A commercially-produced indoor grow tent designed specifically for closet grows can offer you these four benefits over a DIY set-up:

1. Quick Set-up: Attach the aluminum poles in your kit together. Stretch the one-piece tent over the frame you've built. Zip up the sides. And voila! You're ready. Now try to convince me that your 2x4 wood frame will be just as time & cost-effective to build and maintain.

2. Easy Accessibility: Grow tents are designed specifically to accommodate all of the electrical cords and needed ductwork. You'll find numerous tie-in points all over your tent making it easy to set up your specific operation.

3. Optimal Control: Grow tents are designed to easily reflect light and prevent extraneous light from entering during various stages of the growth cycle. You'll be able to establish better control over temperature, humidity and pests.

4. Fast Turn-overs: The walls and floor of your grow tent are designed to be easy to maintain and clean. This'll save you time and energy when cleaning up and getting your next crop ready.

Now the burning question: How much bud can I expect to grow in a 2 x 4 tent?

In order to answer this simple query, we're going to assume that:
Your grow is an average one and that everything went according to plan with few setbacks or difficulties. No major fires, locus infestations or week-long power outages. You've used an average nutrient and you've used them correctly.

A common rule of thumb amongst home growers is to expect upwards of <u>0.5 grams of bud per watt of lighting</u> available. Your light source should penetrate your canopy to a depth of up to 2 feet with the canopy evenly covering the entire 2' x 4' footprint.

So, under ideal, controlled growing conditions, using a 600-watt light source, you can reasonably expect up to 300 grams (10 ounces) of wet bud being produced from your crop. Once dried you'll end up with approximately 1/4 of your original weight or 75 grams (2.7 ounces) of dry bud.

And if you were to pay for this quantity of medicine from a reputable retailer, you could expect to spend anywhere from $525 to $900. Imagine what three grows over the course of a year could save you. Granted you do have the initial cost of setting up your closet grow along with some monthly expenses; however, as you'll soon see, these pale in comparison to what you could save over the course of several years.

Setting up your grow tent with two 450-watt light sources (900 watts in total) strung lengthwise across your tent's footprint should produce about 450 grams wet and 113 grams (4 ounces) dry. This'll be more than plenty of bud to meet most individual's daily medicinal needs over several months.

You'll notice that I didn't mention how many plants you need in order to achieve this goal. In fact, it's not the number of plants you have growing that determines your crop yield, it's your lighting and the surface area of your canopy (tent size) that become the limiting factors.

Choosing the right type of lighting for your grow tent affects yield; as is creating an evenly spread out canopy that covers the entire grow tent footprint.

___

As you can see, quantity is based on the relationship between:
1. Creating a uniform canopy spread across your whole grow tent's footprint.
2. How much light (wattage) is available across that footprint.

This is why it's so important to use growing techniques that produce as even a canopy as possible, while using every nook and cranny of the grow tent footprint so you ensure optimal light penetration. We'll delve into those specific techniques designed to achieve this objective below. Sound good?

As for your bud's quality, this is based on grower talent - your talent. That's why following the current best practices used by the commercial industry makes a whole lot of sense. Wouldn't you agree? We can learn a lot from how cannabis is successfully grown on a large scale and take the best tidbits of advice for our own indoor grow.

What I'm about to share with you, does just that. Years of collective growing experience has been condensed into several easy-to-follow systems to produce the best medicine possible from your home grow initiative. If this doesn't make you want to get on top of the kitchen table and dance the Macarena, I don't know what will.

How much can I expect to spend on equipment?

What follows is a detailed explanation as to how you could set up your closet grow so that you're using the latest technology and best practices while keeping costs manageable. My goal is to have you setting up some of the best equipment available in the market while keeping your total costs under $1000.

This is why I'm going to make specific recommendations as to lighting, humidity control, ventilation systems and temperature control. Using one of my indoor setups as an example, I'll share with you how you could potentially set up your closet grow.

First things first. Before we delve into the nitty gritty of what you should and could purchase, you have a few choices as to where to source your supplies. Going local has always been my focus. And I'm fortunate to live in a city that has one of the largest indoor grow stores and commercial producers of nutrients in the country. When I'm unable to find what I need locally (which is rare) I search for specific items on a large online retail site like Amazon. Most of the links included in the Appendix, that you can check out when you begin researching specific products, are for the online giant Amazon. As previously mentioned, I'm not an Amazon Affiliate and do not personally benefit from any recommendations. What I'm more concerned with is providing you with product links that'll give you a better feel for what is available out in the market. Fair enough?

Even if you're buying local, checking out product reviews and specs online will help you in the decision-making process. Time to check out your home for your kids.

Your Tent:

Investing in a pre-fabricated grow tent is your best option for gaining peace of mind when growing medicine year-round. What we're looking for is a compact, easy-to-setup, grow tent that'll fit in most closets. Like most people, I pulled out my trusty tape measure and measured the inside dimensions of a couple of closets to ensure that what I was going to purchase was going to fit.

The grow tent that I purchased was an iPower 48"x 24"x 60" Grow Tent, which had a 100% water-resistant removable Mylar floor tray for easy cleaning. The tent uses heavy duty zippers and double stitching to protect it from light leaking and ensure durability and long-lasting use. This is a great tent that allows you to control the climate and lighting, so you can grow your plants in any small place safely and easily.

The tear-proof thick tent material with a reflective Mylar interior returns up to 92-97% of your grow light bulbs' light back to your plants. This helps to keep your energy bill low.

What's also important is that this airtight tent keeps your grows contained, prevents odors from leaking out, and stops pests from getting in.

Heavy-duty, all-steel poles, which are rated to handle at least 110 lbs. have been used to build a sturdy frame that'll accommodate all of your equipment needs. The frame is specially finished to ensure smooth installation and safe handling. And no tools are needed for installing the framework.

There are multiple access points around the tent for stringing electrical cords and installing ductwork. These double layer ventilation ducting tubes ensure that no light can penetrate or escape from the tent.

Whether you invest in this model or another, keep some of the above features in mind to help you with the selection process.

Check out this tent by going to Amazon: iPower Grow Tent.
Grow tent budget: $60 - $70 US.

Your Lighting:

Today's lighting technology has allowed indoor growers the capability of growing high-yield cannabis plants using only artificial light. The four most common sources of lighting are:
1. Fluorescent lights.
2. High-intensity discharge (HID) lights.
3. Light-emitting plasma (LEP) lights.
4. Light emitting diodes (LED).

1. Fluorescent lighting is used in a limited capacity in cannabis grows, primarily for raising seedlings or starting clones. The big advantage is that they are inexpensive to purchase and easy to use. The most common sizing's for indoor grows are the T5 and T8 high output bulbs. Fluorescent lights produce the least amount of light of the options listed and must be placed very close (2-4") from the plant to be effective. They'll last about 9000 hours (over 1 year with daily use).

Although great for small plants placed in a clear-plastic, domed, grow tray, there limited versatility for bringing plants to flower makes them a poor choice for most home growers.

2. High-intensity discharge lamps can be loosely grouped according to their composition, as in:
1. Mercury vapor.
2. Metal halide (MH).
3. High-pressure sodium (HP).

These lighting systems require that you hang a reflector that has a HID bulb attached to it. A separate digital ballast (transformer, capacitor and starter) controls the light output as the high-pressure gases enclosed in the clear ceramic arc tube are electrically stimulated.

These systems tend to produce the best quality light but can be costlier in the long run in terms of maintenance and upkeep.

Although popular with large commercial grow ops, HID systems typically have higher energy consumption costs. They tend to produce more heat than other options. Heat dissipation in a small grow space is a concern.

Most high-intensity discharge bulbs last between 12,000 and 24,000 hours (over 2 years with daily use). However, they should be changed annually as they lose some of their light intensity over time.

3. Light-emitting plasma (LEP) lamps generate light by exciting plasma inside a ceramic tube using radio frequency power. They're quiet, energy efficient and rarely fail. This technology is slowly improving as the original models had a hard time delivering the ideal light spectrum to the plants. LEP lights last 30,000 hours (over 4 years with daily use).

The overall light spectrum from LEP lights contains more blue light, which is great for vegetative plant growth that occurs before the flowering and bud development phase. Ideally, we want to have a system that can deliver more blue light during the plant's vegetative growth period and then switch to red spectrum light during flowering. Which brings us to LED lighting.

4. Light-emitting diode (LED) systems are becoming the preferred choice amongst closet growers. LED technology has advanced immensely in the past five years. These lighting systems use solid-state semiconductor energy to produce light.

They are ideal for a home grow as they:
1. Generate less heat than most other technologies.
2. Can be easily plugged into your typical 120 V household plugs, unlike HID lights.
3. Resist damage from external shocks since there are no fragile parts.
4. Are lightweight and compact. Ideal for a closet grow.
5. Have a low operating voltage, thus saving you money on your electrical bill.
6. Can produce light in both the blue and red-light spectrums at the flick of a switch.

LED lights last 50,000 - 100,000 hours (over 5 years of daily use).

We use the Viparspectra Reflector-Series 600W LED Grow Light. It has been developed by indoor growers over many years of careful experimentation and testing.

It comes with an excellent heat dissipation system. The light stays cool - 70% cooler than HID lights. This means that they can be placed closer to your canopy without sun-burning your plants. They're also quiet running, making them less conspicuous in a closet grow.

The Viparspectra 600-Watt model, which has an average power draw of 269W, compares to a 600W HID lamp. The lighting system provides adequate vegetative coverage at a 24" height for a 2 x 4 closet grow. At the flick of a switch you can provide your cannabis plants with the ideal light spectrum based on your plants' growth phase.

Set-up in your grow tent is simple. Just use the ratchet system/ ropes provided to suspend the entire unit in the middle of your tent. Then snake the unit's electrical cord out one of the upper ducting tubes. If your LED unit does not come with a ratchet rope system that allows you to adjust the light's height, you could pick up 2 pairs of **Ledgle ratchet ropes** either locally or from Amazon for about $13.

Along with the LED grow light, you'll want to have the lights set on a simple, manual timer like the Woods 24-hour heavy duty plug-In mechanical timer, which has a 3-prong, grounded outlet. Being a manual timer, it's easy to adjust when your grow lights need to come on and turn off.

LED grow light budget: $170 - $180.
Ratchet rope hangar budget: $13 - $15.
Timer budget: $10 - $12.

What about growing my seedlings, won't the lights be too strong?
Although you could grow your seedlings within your grow tent, using a domed grow tray or "hot house" may be more appropriate. We have a Hydrofarm Jump Start hot house with the heat mat, which has a 7" clear plastic dome with adjustable ventilation.

Whether you're starting from seeds or using clippings (clones), this hot house provides a climate-controlled environment best suited for seedling growth. It's easy to regulate the temperature and humidity within this smaller grow space.

Coupled with a T5 fluorescent bulb, you'll be able to grow your seedlings in a smaller space while keeping your electricity bill low. The 2-foot ViaVolt grow light fixture is lightweight and easy to install. You can use your manual timer destined for your grow tent to deliver the precise duration of light to your seedlings. Plug your T5 light source into the timer. Then, plug the timer and heating mat into a power bar. Easy peasy!

Hot House budget: $35 - $45.
T5 fluorescent light budget: $26 - $36.

Air Purification:

Air ventilation, circulation and purification are essential for any indoor closet grow. Fresh air is critical for optimal plant growth. Think of it this way. In an outdoor growing environment, gentle breezes replace the CO_2 being used by the plant. In an indoor operation, we need to move stale air out of the grow tent and replace it with CO_2-rich air from outside.

The simplest way to do so is to open one of your bottom vents of your grow tent and install an exhaust fan and ducting at the top to draw any stale air out of the tent.

But while we're at it, let's also install a carbon filter that'll eliminate any odors the plants produce, especially during the last few weeks of the flowering phase.

Here's what you'll need to set up a simple ventilation/ purification system. You'll need to invest in:
1. A 6" inline fan designed for home ventilation.
2. A 10-foot section of flexible 6" aluminum ducting. Think clothes dryer ducting.
3. A 6" carbon filter designed for indoor grows.
4. An inline fan air speed adjuster.
5. Three 6" hose clamps for attaching your inline fan, ducting and air filter together.
6. Duct tape to help keep ducting together and airtight.
7. Nylon straps or Ledgle ratchet ropes for suspending the entire ventilation system.
8. Twist or zip ties to keep everything in place.

Here's how you'll set up the ventilation system:
Step 1: Attach a 1-foot section of flexible aluminum ducting to your carbon filter unit with a hose clamp and duct tape.
Step 2: Attach the end of your flexible, aluminum ducting to your inline fan's intake with a 2nd hose clamp and duct tape. Now you'll have your carbon filter attached to your inline fan. Following me so far?

Step 3: Attach a long 6 to 8-foot section of ducting with a 3rd hose clamp to the exhaust port on your inline fan. Now you have your carbon filter attached to your inline fan, which is attached to a lengthy section of ducting that'll snake its way out of your grow tent.

Step 4: Suspend the entire system from straps or ratchet ropes. Keep in mind that you'll be suspending your LED lighting in the centre of the grow tent, so your ventilation system will most likely be suspended just behind the lighting.

Step 5: Snake your long section of ducting out through an upper exhaust tube in the tent.

Step 6. Snake the electrical cord for the inline fan out the same duct tube as your LED lighting system electrical cord.

Step 7. Plug your inline fan into your air speed adjuster. And plug the air speed adjuster cord into an electrical outlet.

What you'll end up with is a suspended carbon filter that draws air from the bottom of your grow tent across the lighting system, through the carbon filter and out of the tent to be recirculated in the room.

Most inline fans are too powerful for a small closet grow, hence the reason for a speed adjuster. We set our air speed adjuster to one of the lowest settings, which does 4 things:

1. Reduces noise.
2. Decreases electricity usage.
3. Maintains a better air flow level for odor control.
4. Reduces the risk of burning out the fan motor.

Along with the ventilation and purification, we also want to ensure that there is an adequate amount of mixing of cooler air from the bottom of the tent with warmer air in the top. This'll be accomplished by setting up a small low wattage 2-speed fan at the height of your canopy.

An easy way to do so is to use zip ties wrapped around an inside vertical tent pole. Set the ties up loose enough so that you can slide the whole unit up and down the pole. I like to have mine set up on the inside right corner of the tent.

I also have my space heater set up on the same side in the back corner with warm air being drawn in from the lower right flap of the tent. The space heater kicks in only when the temperature in the tent drops below 68°F - 70°F. More on this in a moment.

The air is eventually drawn up over the lights and into the carbon filter through the inline fan and exits on the upper right side of the tent through the ducting.

Not only does the circulating fan foster proper mixing of the air, it also helps to strengthen plant stocks. Having stronger stocks, translates into more extensive bud development during flowering. Check out the Vornado Flippi V6 personal air circulator fan for some ideas as to what's out in the market. This fan is energy efficient, drawing less than 30W of power.

Circulating fan budget: $20 - $25.

Besides the small circulating fan described above, we've invested in an iPower fan, filter, ducting combo from Amazon that included a 6" duct inline fan with a 6" carbon filter and 16-foot section of ducting with 2 steel clamps.

Inline fan, carbon filter & ducting budget: $120 to $140.

We also picked up an iPower inline fan air speed adjuster that has 3 speed adjustment settings from 50 - 100%.

Fan air speed adjuster budget: $13 to $15.

Since you may need a 3rd hose clamp, an extra pair of 6" steel hose clamps will set you back about $6. And 4 Ledgle grow light ratchet rope hangars are about $13.

Visualizing how these components are set up as you read through this material may be challenging. There are many YouTube videos that'll show you how you could set things up should you need a visual reference. Just head on over to You Tube and type "marijuana grow tent setup" in the search bar.

I've mentioned setting up a small space heater in your tent as a precaution for when the tent might cool down too much. Let's take a look at how we're going to control both humidity and temperature in the following section.

Humidity and Temperature Control:

As previously mentioned, humidity and temperature along with lighting determines how much CBD-rich medicine your cannabis plants are going to produce over a typical 4-month grow cycle.

During the early stages of growth, seedlings are delicate, requiring relatively higher levels of humidity in the range of 60 - 80%. And they'll thrive when the air temperature hovers between 70°F - 80°F (ideally, around 78°F). Later on, during the tail end of bud development which occurs during the flowering phase, your plants are going to respond better with a lower level of both humidity (40 - 50%) and temperature (ideally, around 72°F). But how do we best monitor these parameters and maintain an optimal range for sustained growth?

The first part of the answer lies in how to effectively monitor both relative humidity and temperature during all phases of the growth cycle.

We like to use a compact, battery-operated (one AAA battery) ThermoPro indoor humidity and temperature monitor for our grows. It can be easily moved and set up in any growing environment, whether it be a small domed, seedling, hot house or your grow tent. It will display the current, lowest and highest levels of temperature and humidity over a time period. I like to reset the monitor every day, so that I know immediately if I have to adjust any parameters in my grow. This is especially critical during seedling development.

Humidity/ temperature monitor budget: $8 to $10.

The second part of the answer lies in what specific devices could we use to create those ideal environmental factors.

Here are two simple solutions. Once again, I'm using Amazon's supply chain to illustrate what you could potentially invest in that has worked out for us. If you're buying local, look for comparable designs and price points. ***Solution #1***: You can purchase a compact humidifier for under $60 like the Taotronics cool mist humidifier, which comes with a 1-gallon reservoir, built in timer and low power consumption of about 30W.

Humidifier budget: $43 to $50.

A humidifier allows you to precisely regulate the level of moisture your plants receive over the course of the various phases of growth. Higher humidity to begin with and lower levels as the flower sites develop during the tail end of your flowering phase.

I don't like to rely solely on the unit's built in humidity sensors to keep me abreast as to how the relative humidity is holding up. I like to tweak the humidifier settings based on feedback from my portable indoor humidity and temperature monitor. Keep in mind that we're going to have to be space conscious in setting up our grow. Your plants should occupy the majority of your tent's footprint, not your humidifier, fan or space heater.

Solution #2: To maintain a proper temperature level for our personal "northern" grows, we have a Honeywell heat bud ceramic heater which kicks out 170W and 250W of power based on the 2 settings built into the unit. If you live in a region where air conditioners are not the norm, or should you reside in the far reaches of Canada amongst the polar bears, then spending under $25 on a heater ensures that you're potentially growing the best medicine you can. This compact heater or a similar sized model should provide just enough heat to regulate the temperature range in your tent. It's a good space heater for small areas, like at your feet if you're by a desk. However, this particular unit is <u>insufficient</u> in size to heat a small room. And that's probably a good thing. We don't want to bake our precious babies. And, we would like to keep our energy consumption footprint small.

Compact space heater budget: $17 to $20.

And how do you regulate the heat in your grow tent? Glad you asked. You can regulate this heater better by using a thermostat controller.

We have our space heater plugged into an Inkbird outlet thermostat controller. The controller is a small, programmable unit with a temperature probe. The long wire probe can be fished through one of your grow tent's ducting sleeves, while the actual controller resides close to your tent. Position the probe just above your canopy to get the most accurate indication as to how your plants are faring.

The controller is then plugged into an electrical outlet (power strip). The cord on your compact heater would also be fished through a tent sleeve and plugged into your thermostat controller. Now, when the temperature in your tent drops below a specific set point, your space heater kicks in shutting off when it reaches your upper setting.

We can easily program low and high temperature settings of 70°F and 78°F to ensure that the plants are not subjected to wide temperature swings of more than 10 degrees. An important point to keep in mind. Too much stress to the plant, whether it be big fluctuations in temperature, humidity or light result in slower and possibly poorer quality grows. Hence, the reason why incorporating some simple, inexpensive devices to better control your grow tent's environment and ultimately the quantity and quality of CBD medicine makes a whole lot of "cents".

Thermostat controller budget: $35 to $50.

What if it gets really cold in my grow tent?
Great question, especially if you're growing in a northern clime, you've already set up a space heater AND you're still finding the grow environment too cold.

Here are some practical tips to keeping your plants warmer:
1. Elevate your pots onto a closed celled foam pad, similar to what you would use on a tent-camping trip. This'll help stop heat loss through the root zone of your pots.

2. Alternatively, you could place a seedling heating mat often sold with domed plastic hot houses under or near your plant(s).
3. Loosely wrap the sides of your pots with an insulating foam that has some breathability. You don't want to cut off all of the air flow, just the cold air from constantly hitting the sides.
4. Try to increase the overall room temperature if possible. This may be a no-brainer for some. However, not all closet growers have control over the amount of heat reaching their room, especially if you're sharing a common heating system as in an apartment, condo or possibly basement suite.
5. Possibly invest in a slightly larger portable heater that you could place closer to the grow tent's intake flap. Look for one that won't crank out more than 1500 Watts of power. You'll need to plug this baby into an outlet separate from your closet grow outlet or you'll be constantly blowing the electrical breaker.
6. Also keep your bags or containers of growing medium off a cold floor and warm it up before use if you're keeping it in a cool shed or room.
7. Consider running your grow lights at night when its cooler. In some jurisdictions, this may even save you some money on the cost of the electricity you'll be paying. Wouldn't that be the cat's meow?

Do I need a dehumidifier?

While a de-humidifier unit helps to better regulate humidity levels, especially at the end of your grow, it's probably not an essential investment. We have a Bionaire BD10 series digital dehumidifier that's great for small rooms. We use ours to draw moisture out of the room in the last 2 weeks of bud development and to help during the week-long drying period. Pro Breeze has an inexpensive mini dehumidifier that's compact and portable.

Dehumidifier budget: $80 to $100. Optional.

Electrical Basics:

Being a discrete closet grow, you'll be able to use just one standard 120-volt service wall plug for your set-up. Most wall plugs are 15-amp circuits, meaning that you'll be able to draw approximately 1440W of continuous power before triggering a breaker (1800 watts less 20%). And since our final set-up will only draw a maximum of 800W, we're golden.

As far as power bars and extension cords, you'll need at a minimum, you'll probably want to use a 12-outlet grounded power bar with surge protection, so you don't fry any components, especially if you have a "dirty" electrical supply. Although you won't need all 12 outlets, having them spaced out more than a 6-outlet unit makes it easier to plug in components like your manual light timer and space heater. Along with this, count on 3 extension cords to make it easier to hook everything up.

As well, when you are setting everything up initially, ensure that you unplug from the power source first. Or, if everything is being plugged into your power bar, turn it off. Work backwards, as outlined below, when installing electrical components.

Here's what I've done in this "example closet grow" set-up:
1. Power Source -> Power Bar:
I have an extension cord connecting my power source to the power bar, which is placed in close proximity to where your tent will be and preferably at the height of your tent. You may even consider placing your cording on top of your tent depending on whether your tent will support the weight or not. Much of my cording is on top of the tent, which gives me easy access.

Check out the Belkin 12-outlet power strip surge protector on a site like Amazon to get some idea as to what might work. You should be able to pick up a power strip for $18 - $22.

2. Inline Fan -> Speed Controller -> Power Bar:
Then, I've connected my inline fan to my speed controller, which is plugged into the power bar.

3. LED Lights -> Manual Timer -> Power Bar:

Next, I've connected my LED lights to the manual timer, which controls when the lights turn on and off. This unit is plugged into the power bar.

4. Desk Fan -> Power Bar:

My desk fan is also plugged into my power bar. However, for greater flexibility as to where in the tent you'll position the fan, consider using a short extension cord. A 6' - 8' cord could be adequate for your specific situation.

5. Humidifier -> Extension Cord -> Power Bar:

For both the humidifier and space heater, I like to have them both set up on extension cords. This allows me the option of easily removing each unit without disturbing the grow or becoming frustrated struggling with the cords. I can run the extension cord between the inside wall of the tent and the waterproof floor catch basin that comes with the tent. Out of sight, out of mind.

6. Space Heater -> Extension Cord -> Temperature Controller -> Power Bar:

The same situation applies here as for the humidifier. Usually your heater and desk fan will be set up on the opposite end of your tent as your humidifier. I have my humidifier on the left side and the heater/ fan on the right side. The key is to maintain easy access to your heater while having any cording discretely tucked away.

What type of extension cord should I be using?

As for which type of extension cord you should consider using, be aware that electricity flowing through wire creates heat. And heat is wasted power. Using a 14-guage wire for a 120-volt outlet that has a grounded (3-prong) wire connection is important. Using a 16 or 18-gauge wire forces too much power through the cord. This causes the wire to heat up and also causes a drop in voltage (pressure), which means less efficiency from your lights. And if you need to run an extension cord for more than 50 feet, use a 12-guage cord.

A 14-guage, 15-foot, heavy duty, grounded (3-prong) extension cord is about $14. Your budget for a power bar and extension cords can vary greatly depending on both your needs and preferences. For a good quality set-up of 3 extension cords along with a power bar expect to budget $65.

Let's Recap.

We now have our self-contained grow tent set up with an energy-efficient LED lighting system. Our inline fan draws cool air from the bottom of our tent mixing it with warmer air located by the lighting system and pulling this and any odors through a carbon filter out through the ducting into the room to be re-circulated. We also have a small fan set up to gently bow air across our cannabis plants reducing the chance of developing any molds or mildew while strengthening the plant's stalks.

Let's check out what we've invested in so far for setting up our stealth grow. So far, we've accounted for:
1. Our 4' x 2' x 5' tent designed specifically for indoor grows.
2. A doomed seedling hot house, heating mat and T5 fluorescent light source.
3. A carbon filter that is hooked up to an inline fan and ducting.
4. A 600-watt LED lighting system on adjustable pulleys and attached to a 24-hour timer.
5. A small portable fan discreetly tucked into one corner of the tent.
6. A humidifier set up during the seedling and vegetative growth phases.
7. A heater set up in case we need to maintain our ideal temperature ranges.
8. And we're accurately monitoring and controlling temperature and relative humidity.

We've spent between $595 and $680 so far in building the infrastructure for our grow op. Well under our $1000 total projected budget. Now, we need to address both the growing medium and nutritional needs of our babies. Time to boot, scoot and boogie. Well ... maybe not.

Four optimal growth factors:

Optimal growth of your plants is based on the interaction of the following four key elements:

1. Moist roots. Roots flourish when they are moist at all times and die when they dry out.

2. Oxygenation. Roots take in oxygen. The more oxygen that is readily available to your plant's root system the more developed the growth.

3. Essential Nutrients. Roots take up nutrients and deliver them to the rest of the plant. Providing your plants with easy access to the right combinations of essential nutrients helps your plants thrive and produce the quality medicine you desire.

4. Managing pH. Nutrient uptake depends on the pH of the growing medium. When the pH rises above 7.0 or drops below 5.5 the availability of certain essential nutrients diminishes. Providing nutrients with the correct pH level ensures optimal uptake and growth. Maintaining a pH between 6.2 and 6.5 is in the "sweet" zone for most growing mediums and cannabis strains.

We'll be addressing each of these key elements when we look at the specifics as to how to grow your plants in an ideal environment. For now, let's look at what your choices are for growing mediums. The three most common growing mediums that home growers like yourself use are:
1. Soil
2. Coco coir.
3. Hydroponics.

1. Soil: Soil is the most common growing medium used by closet growers. Since it is the most natural growing medium that the plant is used to in the wild, it tends to be the easiest medium to use when starting out.

Look for all organic potting soil like Black Gold should you be growing in a natural soil medium. Going organic allows you to conduct your grow in hopefully a healthier environment. You could also mix 20% Perlite into your soil. Perlite is specially treated inert volcanic glass that resists soil compaction and encourages aeration. It's ideal for high humidity indoor plant grows like cannabis.

The biggest benefit of soil is that you're dealing with a natural growing medium that already contains some of the nutrients required for sustaining plant grow. pH tends to be easier to manage when using a properly amended and composted soil. It's an easy growing medium for beginners to initially work with.

On the flip side, soil often carries pests into the growing area, which you'll need to deal with from the get-go. No need to fret about this. I'll show you 3 effective ways of dealing with some of the most common pests that can enter the grow area.

2. Coco Coir: Coco coir is an inert growing medium made of fibrous coconut husks. Coco coir is a great soilless growing medium for cannabis. It acts like soil in that you'll keep your plants in pots filled with the growing medium and then simply water and feed your babies with nutrient water.

Unlike soil, which tends to hold onto or retain excess water, coco coir helps prevent over or under-watering since it drains well and re-hydrates easily. Also, the medium has a lighter texture that lets it hold onto more oxygen which is ideal for root development and prevents waterlogging. This tends to promote faster and healthier root development. It is an ideal host material for hosting beneficial, root-enhancing microbes, which help to increase growth rates and bud development.

The four biggest advantages of coco coir are that:
1. It doesn't make a good home for insects. Coco coir tends to dry out on top, so you'll have fewer problems with fungus gnats.
2. You get to precisely control the type and amount of nutrients you'll be adding throughout the entire grow.

3. It's difficult to over-water and is more forgiving should you over-feed your darlings since it doesn't hold or store nutrient or organic salts as much as soil.
4. Being an inert medium, you can use both hydroponic and organic nutrient formulations.

The downside is that you'll need to provide nutrients from the beginning, since this is an inert growing medium, unlike soil. You'll also need to add a small amount of Cal-Mag (calcium-magnesium) supplement along with your other nutrients as coco coir tends to need more. Granted, there are companies like Advanced Nutrients (USA) and Diablo Nutrients (Canada) that have accounted for this deficiency in their formulations.

3. Hydroponics: Hydroponics is a soilless growing medium that only uses nutrient-rich water for sustaining plant growth. It's very effective in delivering just the right amount of nutrients to your plants. And since the plant's root system is constantly bathed in water, the plant doesn't need to spend a lot of energy developing an elaborate network. In fact, hydro will save the average grower about 2 weeks during the vegetative growth phase because of this.

The downside of hydro is the cost of the initial set-up and the steep learning curve in figuring out the optimum growing conditions. It can be a bit more labor intensive than other growing mediums.

Growing in coco coir - What you need to know:

Coco coir is my preferred medium for growing because of the four advantages previously mentioned. Sure, it's a little more challenging than growing in soil. However, it allows me greater control as to what nutrients to add during the various phases of the growing cycle.

Here are some tips on how to optimize your grow in coco coir:
Tip #1: Buy the best. Coco coir comes in various forms such as compressed bricks, loose fiber, or mixed with Perlite. Look for clean, golden-brown fibers void of clumps or fine powder. Brick coco coir is usually the least expensive, but harder to work with than loose-fiber coco coir. Ensure that the coco coir has been rinsed prior to packaging so that any salts have been flushed out of the fibers.

Tip #2: Rinse and Test. Before using any coco coir in a grow, take the time to rinse the fibers with clean, neutral pH water. I like to rinse my loose-fiber coco coir with reverse osmosis water that is slightly alkaline (pH = 6.0 - 6.5). Simply, place your coco coir in a large 3 to 5-gallon bucket of clean water, stir it up with your hand for a couple of minutes, grab handfuls of fiber and squeeze the excess water out of it, while transferring the material into another container for a 2nd rinse. I like to test the final run-off to ensure that the salt content is less than 400 ppm (parts per million) with a TDS meter.

Tip #3: Use reverse osmosis (RO) water. Coco coir reacts quickly to salts and contaminants because it has no chemical or physical properties that interact with water and whatever is in it, unlike soil or hydroponic grows. For this reason, it's better to start with pH neutral water containing no impurities - hence the importance of using RO or distilled water.

Tip #4: Use nutrient systems designed for cannabis grows. Both Advanced Nutrients (USA) and Diablo Nutrients (Canada) have an array of products to get the most out of your grows. The challenge with coco coir is that it tends to lock-out (prevent the uptake of) magnesium and calcium crucial for photosynthesis and bud development in the flowering stage. Adding small quantities of Cal-Mag for each feeding helps. Or, you can use products specially formulated with this in mind.

Whether you decide to go with an "all-natural" grow in soil or venture into coco coir, you'll need a certain amount of growing medium for your closet grow. Expect to purchase between 3 and 4 cubic feet of growing medium at your local gardening store or plant nursery.

A bag or compressed brick of Coco Coir can be purchased online or locally for $15 - $20.

Soil/ coco budget: $20 - $40.

What about pots?

There are three main types of pots used in indoor cannabis grows, namely:

1. Plastic Pots.
2. Smart Pots.
3. Air Pots.

1. Regular Plastic Pots.

The least expensive container option is a plastic pot, which has a hole or holes at the bottom for drainage, along with a saucer or tray to capture runoff water.

Any gardening store will carry an assortment of pot sizes with the 3-gallon and 5-gallon pots being the most practical pot for an indoor closet grow.

The main advantage, besides cost, of using plastic pots is that it is a solid container, and this helps keep the growing medium from drying out too quickly.

The downside, is just that, possibly retaining too much water and causing root damage to your plants. There are two better alternatives to plastic pots, which will address the common problem of overwatering your babies. These are Smart pots and Air pots.

2. Smart Pots.

A smart pot is a flexible plant container that has been made completely out of a stiff, breathable, porous fabric.

They are usually wider and shorter than other pot designs, making them well-suited for a closet grow. The wide base of a Smart pot makes these pots very stable. On the flip side, being wider, you'll need to take this into account when planning the layout of your grow tent.

You'll need to purchase large saucers to capture water run-off since these pots don't come with run-off collection trays. This means that you will need to accommodate the extra room for the saucers in your footprint as well.

The biggest advantage of the Smart pot system is that more oxygen is delivered to the roots than a regular pot. They prevent your plants from becoming root-bound and needing to be transplanted to a new container, which causes a temporary shock to the plants. This is accomplished by air-pruning roots from the sides, which stops the roots from wrapping around the edges of your container and choking your plant.

Having porous sides means that Smart pots make it difficult to over-water your plants. However, it also means you may end up watering more often. This can be avoided by using a larger final-size container. Many home growers have had success with 5-gallon Smart pots. We usually have three 5-gallon pots set up comfortably in our 2' x 4' tent. These pots sit on deep 14" plastic saucers, which collect any run-off.

Alternatively, you could set up five 3-gallon pots in the same tent space, using a 10" saucer for each pot. Just keep in mind, that you may need to be more vigilant in your watering regime with the smaller pot size.

The Smart Pot 5-gallon soft-sided fabric garden plant container comes in a 5-pack set, which ends up being less expensive than buying them individually.

Smart Pot Budget: $29 - $32.

3. Air Pots.
An air pot is a solid plastic container with multiple, tiny holes on the sides that function similar to a fabric Smart pot. Water is allowed to seep out the sides when watering.

They tend to be taller and thinner than a regular plastic pot container, so it may be possible to put more plants in a smaller space as long as you have the height. However, a narrower base means that the air pots tend to be less stable on the ground since they're easier to tip over.

We suggest using a set of three 5-gallon air pots or a set of five 3-gallon ones for a small closet grow.

As with the Smart pot, you'll find that more oxygen is delivered to the roots than a regular plastic pot and overwatering becomes less of an issue.

The one downside may be the cost, as this is the costliest alternative of the three mentioned.

MaXX yield 5-gallon air root pruning pots come in a 6-pack set should you be picking them up on a site like Amazon.
Air Pot Budget: $60 - $65.

Hydrofarm 14" Water Drip Tray.
These 14" heavy plastic round saucer water drip trays are designed for plant growing and come in a set of 10. They work well with a 5-gallon pot system. You'll be able to set up 3 trays and Smart Pots into your 2'x 4' grow tent and still have room for a humidifier and space heater, if needed. Keep in mind, that there are many brands of drip trays to choose from as well as local options to consider. And do you need a set of 10? No. However, you can check out options online and then purchase the quantity you might need locally.

Water Drip Tray Budget: $15 - $18.

Let's summarize our pot selection:
Your plants will grow faster in either Smart or Air pots, in part because plant roots get plenty of access to oxygen. Keep in mind that we want to avoid having your plants become root-bound, in which the roots wrap around the edge of the container choking the plant.

Your plants are protected from becoming overwatered in Smart pots or Air pots. The air from the side helps make sure your plants always have plenty of oxygen, so your plants don't drown.

However, plants in these pots need to be watered about twice as often as regular plastic containers since the grow medium is constantly drying out from the sides. We'll address this concern when we look at feeding and watering regimes. Moving on to SCRoGing.

What the heck is SCRoGing?

Besides our growing medium and pots, you'll also want to spend a few dollars on a **SCRoG (screen of green) string trellis net**. No, it's not something you'll be using to trap fish to be eventually composted and added to your grows.

Since we want to use as much canopy space as your tent's footprint will allow, a lightweight netting will give us the ability to control how each branch grows in the tent.

The technique we'll be using to achieve optimal coverage of your tent space with an even canopy for maximum light exposure is called SCRoGing. We'll be training each of your plants during the grow to spread out under a net set to help contain each branch. Remember, the maximum yield you can produce out of your grow op is dependent on two major factors - light intensity spread out across the tent and having an even canopy of green making optimal use of your floor space.

You can attach the SCRoG net with plastic ties or better yet create a lightweight frame out of a 12-foot section of 1" PVC pipe and 4 elbow connectors. Yes, you will need to use a little MacGyver ingenuity to get'er done. However, having a simple, lightweight frame makes it easier to adjust the height of your SCRoG should need be. Something to consider setting up for a few bucks, right?

What I've done for a 2' x 4' tent space is cut two 2'-sections and two 4'-foot sections of PVC pipe. Then I slide the four elbow joints onto the ends creating a frame. Once the frame is set up, I attach a section of SCRoG netting to the frame with nylon cable ties. You could even use duct tape in a pinch. Once assembled, this whole unit can be easily slid into the tent and attached to the four corners of your tent with nylon cable ties. You'll use this contraption from the beginning of the flowering phase of your kids onwards.

SCRoG Trellis Net Budget: $12 - $15.

How important are nutrients in the grow cycle?

Nutrients support quality growth in your plants and help to optimize your crop yield. During the process of photosynthesis, cannabis uses water being pulled into the plant from the roots along with carbon dioxide being pulled in through the leaves to produce sugars that increase plant growth. Adding the appropriate nutrients helps the plant transport essential enzymes, hormones and sugars up into the plant where it is used to increase growth. As light energy is being converted into chemical energy the plant transpires emitting water and oxygen through its leaves.

Nutrients are important to help the plant transport substances around that build cellular structures. However, don't get caught up in the hype surrounding one commercially available nutritional product or supplement over another. If there was one magic formula that could get you incredible yields, wouldn't there already be farmers using this magic formula to consistently produce humungous crops? It's just not the case.

The correct amount of nutrients is the correct amount of nutrients you can feed the plant while still getting optimal yield. Nutrients are primarily salts. Your plants will only absorb what they can handle. Anything else builds up in the plant becoming toxic to the plant. Too much salt buildup in the growing medium prevents water from rising up into the plant. The reverse actually happens with water flowing down to the roots in an attempt to remedy this toxic state. Eventually, the plant leaves become dehydrated turning yellow or brown in the process and photosynthesis is slowed down.

With this in mind, let's take a look at a few basic nutrient systems that'll get you started in the right direction. Now, keep in mind that each of these manufacturers has an extensive list of supplements to choose from. Avoid getting caught up in the hype by buying everything that's available. Start slowly, building upon the basics you'll require to have a successful grow.

Feeding your darlings the right way:

Most fertilizers appropriate for growing cannabis are based on a 3-bottle system. There's usually a Grow formulation designed for abundant green growth. Then, there's a Bloom formulation used during flowering. And, there's usually a third micro-nutrient formulation that's used throughout all of the main growth phases to increase root development and nutrient uptake. Here are 4 possibilities to consider:

1. Diablo.

I personally use the Diablo product line of nutrients manufactured in British Columbia, since they have been designed by researchers and growers - for growers. And we've all heard about the reputation of BC Bud, right?

Check out their product line at: Diablo Nutrients. Their basic nutrient system is the Grow, Micro and Bloom formulations. These will get you started on the right path.

2. Advanced Nutrients.

Advanced Nutrients is another Canadian-based company out of British Columbia. Their team of researchers has been around since the late 90's creating, testing and optimizing their nutrient system geared for the medical cannabis grower.

Check out their line of Coco Base Nutrients on Amazon. Their Coco Base Nutrients Sensi Grow and Bloom are specially formulated for coco coir users. They use a pH Perfect technology that eliminates trouble-some pH levels. The combo pack contains two 1-Liter (32 ounce) bottles.

3. FoxFarm.

FoxFarm has a 3-pack nutrient system that'll meet the primary nutritional needs of your cannabis plants. The formulations tend to be geared more towards plant growers in general, as opposed to cannabis cultivars. Something to consider. The 3-pack set of 32-ounce bottles includes: Big Bloom, Grow Big and Tiger Bloom liquid fertilizer.

4. General Hydroponics.

General Hydroponics Flora 3-pack nutrient system is also an alternative product line to consider using. Once again, the formulations tend to be more generic for plant growth.

Base Nutrient Budget: $40 - $60.

If you're growing in neutral coco coir, consider using a product like Botanicare Cal-Mag as a plant supplement. The coco coir naturally holds onto calcium and magnesium. Depending on the nutrient system that you're going to use, add small quantities of this supplement to prevent any lockout of other nutrients.

Cal-Mag Budget: $16 - $25.

Two optional supplements to consider purchasing are:
1. Bud Candy from Advanced Nutrients. It provides an assortment of sugars and nutrients for the plant that help to bring out the natural sweetness in the bud.

Bud Candy Budget: $24 - $28.

2. Great White Mycorrhizae. Mycorrhizae are natural fungi that work symbiotically with the root structures of plants. The fungi help wards off disease and insects while promoting root growth. A small 1oz. package of powder is all you'll need to get started. Add the mycorrhizae to your pots anytime you transplant your precious babies.

Mycorrhizae Budget: $13 - $15.

Monitoring your nutrient additions:

How much is enough? And when should I be feeding my babies? Two excellent questions Watson.

To best monitor and control how much nutrition your plants are receiving (nutrient concentration levels) and what pH level is going to provide you with adequate nutrient uptake, I recommend investing in inexpensive pH and TDS meters.

123

For example, the Vivosun pH & TDS meter combo, can be purchased on Amazon for under $20. These inexpensive pen-type meters are easy-to-use and accurate enough for any indoor closet grow. They'll be a vital part of your success in growing a CBD-rich crop over and over again.

The pH meter will be used to gauge how acidic or alkaline your nutrient solution is. Ideally, we're looking for a slightly acidic formulation in the range of 6.0 to 6.5. This pH range seems to work well for most soil or soilless growing situations.

The TDS meter is used to determine how concentrated each feeding is, so as not to under or over-feed your plants. More on the feeding regime for you plants later in this section. For now, what's important to understand is that these meters measure the electrical conductivity of the salts and chemicals being added to your feeding formulations. A TDS meter often provides information in parts per million (ppm) and electrical conductivity (EC). Most of the examples given in this book are in ppm. Should you like to convert to EC units, simply divide your ppm by 500. For example, a ppm of 1000 is equal to 1000/500 = 2.0 EC. Quick and simple.

pH and TDS Meter Budget: $17 - $20.

I also like to pick up some pH test paper to periodically check my pH meter's readings. An inexpensive roll of test strips ensures that you're not killing your plants because your pH levels are out of wack.

Along with your pH meter, you'll want to pick up a couple of helpful kits. One is for accurately calibrating your pH meter. The General Hydroponics pH 4.01 & pH 7.0 calibration solution kit will do the trick. Use these 2 solutions in order to accurately calibrate your pH meter each month or so.

pH Calibration Kit Budget: $15 - $18.

Once you've measured your final nutrient formulation for your feed, you'll need to adjust the pH level so that it falls within an optimal range for plant growth. This can be done with something like the General Hydroponics pH Up & Down kit.

Each 8-ounce bottle of pH down uses food grade phosphoric acid to lower pH to the desired level. Up contains potassium carbonate and potassium silicate. These chemicals, in the quantities you'll be using, will have no adverse effects on you or the medicine you'll be growing.

pH Up & Down Budget: $16 - $20.

Something else to consider picking up, is a soil moisture meter that'll help you assess how dry or moist your growing medium is becoming.

Most garden shops carry simple soil moisture meters. You can easily measure the soil's moisture content by plugging in the probe into the soil. No electricity or plug outlet is needed. I use one to assess how dry the first inch of my growing medium is in comparison to the bottom. The scale gives you a "general" idea as to how much moisture is being retained, thus allowing you to know when to best schedule your next watering or feeding.

Soil Moisture Meter Budget: $10 - $12.

So far you have a pretty good idea as to what two recommended types of containers to use, along with several options for nutrient systems to consider using and how to monitor what you're feeding your plants. Let's take a look at four proactive (rather than reactive) ways to control pests. Using a proactive approach in controlling for bug infestations (and every grower has to deal with those pesky little creatures at some point in time) is less invasive and costly than having to treat your plants and potting medium with a less than desirable chemical option.

Effective pest control:

Here's a simple proactive approach to dealing with bugs trying to eat your crop:
1. Ensure that any fruit you bring into your home has been washed thoroughly should you be leaving it on the kitchen counter. Nasty little bugs and their eggs may be hitching a ride into your home just waiting for you to grow some delicious cannabis plants for them to munch on.

2. Invest in yellow sticky paper like the Trapro 20-Pack dual-sided yellow sticky traps. These yellow-colored sticky sheets are great for trapping flying plant insects like fungus gnats, aphids, whiteflies and leaf-miners. I set a couple of sheets up in my grow tent to ensure that no bug infestation will ruin my crops. Also, place them near other household plants or fruit to keep them in check.

Yellow Sticky Trap Budget: $10 - $12.

3. Nutrilife SM-90 plant growth fertilizer is an organic composition that stimulates new and better root growth. It increases the speed of moisture penetration in growing mediums. SM-90 also helps contain gnats who take up residence in your growing medium. It can be used for systemic (root) feeding to prevent problems, as well as used as a foliar spray to stop bug attacks in their tracks. The main ingredients of SM-90 are coriander and canola oil. The sweet smell of coriander helps mask offensive odors coming from organic products containing bat guano or the like.

SM-90 Budget: $21 - $25.

4. TanLin is a safe and effective remedy against maggots eating your plant's root system and evolving into fungus gnats. Adding just a few drops from the 1 ounce bottle each time you feed your plants helps to keep insects in check. I use this product as an initial treatment any time that I introduce new growing medium into my grow operation.

TanLin Budget: $44 - $50.

Additional investment considerations:

1. Disposable Medical Grade Gloves.
Nitrile Gloves that are medical grade, powder and latex rubber free come in handy when handling delicate plants, as well as during harvest and drying. A box of 100 can be purchased locally for under $8.

2. Isopropyl alcohol.
A simple yet effective way to sterilize tools is with isopropyl alcohol, which can be purchased locally for under $7 a 16-ounce (1 Liter) bottle. Alcohol also easily dissolves the resin that collects on instruments and your hands when harvesting your crop.

3. Mars Hydro LED Glasses. Eye protection is paramount when using any type of lighting system in a grow tent. The green lenses are designed to protect your eyes under HPS, MH and LED lighting systems. They do reduce the eyestrain and alleviate the pain from harsh lighting.

Protective Eyeglasses Budget: $15 - $20.

4. Pruning Snips like the Tabor pruning shears offer a pointed, thin blade that reaches into the tightest spaces. When shaping your cannabis plants during the grow and for the final harvest and processing you'll want a precision cutting tool that's easy to handle for potentially long periods of time. This is where having needle-nosed trimmers comes in very handy.

Pruning Shears Budget: $10 - $15.

5. Individual plastic drinking cups like the Solimo disposable plastic cups from Amazon are great for starting seedlings. Not to mention having a brew-ski while working on your plants or after a successful harvest.

Use your pruning shears or scissors to snip 3 small drainage holes evenly spaced out on the bottom corner of your cups. This'll allow water and feeding solution to drain from the cups that'll be filled with your growing medium. These 18-ounce drinking cups are easy to find locally. Just remember not to use any of these cups after for that slightly chilled pint of Amber Ale.

Solo Plastic Drinking Cup Budget: $4 - $5.

6. Nylon Cable Ties come in handy when you want to set up your equipment in your grow tent, such as your electrical cording, SCRoG net and possibly for your plants. You can pick up an assortment of sizes to meet your needs at any hardware store. They're usually sold in packs of 50 to 300. I like to get longer ones that I'm able to trim to the final desired size. Just wrap the tie around your object(s), pull one end of the tie through the other and cinch it tight. Voila! Done.

Nylon Cable Ties Budget: $5 - $10.

These additional investment considerations will cost you about 50 bucks to purchase. And some of these items or similar ones may already be lurking in your home.

Nice to have considerations:

1. Pocket microscope.
The Carson MicroBrite Plus 60x - 120x power LED lighted pocket microscope is what we use when we want to investigate any leaf discolorations, identify male plants in the grow tent and to help us determine the optimal time to harvest our buds based on the trichome development.

Pocket Microscope Budget: $13 - $15.

2. Coffeevac Storage Canister.
The Coffeevac one-pound, vacuum-sealed, coffee container is ideal for storing your bud. The canister produces a partial vacuum, which keeps your bud fresher for longer. Something to consider, right?

Coffeevac Budget: $15 - $18.

3. Ona Gel Odor Neutralizer.

Ona Pro gel in a 1-quart size neutralizes odors naturally. We use this gel in our grow room to eliminate any odors when we have to open up the grow tent for longer periods of time for any reason, especially as the plants start to produce big, aromatic, resinous buds. This is an effective solution for controlling cannabis odors temporarily in a room. The company even has a fan unit that you can place on top of the gel container to help dissipate all of that steamy goodness contained within.

Ona Gel Budget: $25 - $28.

4. Precision Pocket Scale.

A precision jewelry pocket scale that's accurate to 0.01 g. will meet your future needs should you be weighing out small quantities of your final product. Look for a back-lit LCD display that's easy to read.

Precision Pocket Scale Budget: $10 - $12.

5. Compassionate Analytics CBD / THC test kits provide a simple, inexpensive and relatively accurate analysis of how much CBD or THC is contained in your cannabis buds. If you're going to be creating some of your own CBD-rich products, having an idea as to the starting concentration gives you better control as to the dosing levels you can expect from your products.

CBD Test Kit Budget: $50.

6. Bubble Bags from the industry leader "BubbleBagDude" sells a 4-bag set of extraction bags for making water/ ice kief (more on that in Phase 8: Making CBD-Rich Products). Recall that kief is the resinous material high in cannabinoids that's left over after any green plant material has been separated out. Four 5-gallon bags come in a set of 220, 120, 73 and 40 microns for extracting pure cannabis resin. You'll even get a 25-micron pressing screen along with a convenient storage bag. Even though I've listed this under optional investments, producing your own kief opens up a whole world of possibilities as to how to use your CBD-rich extract. Something worth investing in, right?

Set of Bubble Bags Budget: $25 - $28.

8. Wet/dry vacuum.
A small 5-gallon capacity wet-dry vacuum comes in handy for cleaning up spills and when you need to flush your pots with clean water a week or so just before harvest. We've found this to be the easiest way of removing the overflow from your water drip trays. You should be able to find a vacuum locally for under $65.

So, what's the bottom line, R.J.?

Of course, you need not invest in all of these various products in order to set up a successful closet grow operation. However, down the road you may wish to invest in certain items that'll make it easier to consistently produce quality medicine.

So, where are we at in our total budget? We've invested between $595 and $680 in setting up our tent infrastructure, along with the environmental control. We've purchased pots and growing medium to the tune of $85 - $100. A starter nutrient combo pack and monitoring devices will run us between $58 to $70. A proactive pest control system will be about $75 to $85. And some basic tools will cost about $55. At this point you'll have invested between $870 and $990.

Granted, you may have several of these or similar items kicking around your home, which of course will lower your overall set-up costs.

How long should I expect my supplies to last?

By buying quality from the get-go, you can expect a longer life out of your equipment. This initial equipment set-up should give you more than two years of pleasure. As for your nutrient and chemical supplies, expect roughly the same period of time before having to re-stock.

Recall that our four primary goals for our closet grow are:
1. Being stealthy and discreet from preying eyes.
2. Having a small footprint so that we can grow in a small space - like a closet.
3. Being easy to manage on a day-to-day basis.
4. Being cost effective in producing our own quality medicine.

So, how much power will this closet grow use on average each month?

Granted your power consumption will vary over the course of a 4-month grow cycle. However, we can determine an average monthly power consumption cost based on the closet grow set-up I've just described above.

During the vegetative phase of plant grow, which lasts about 4 weeks you can expect to use less than 8kW hours per day or 240kW over the course of the month. This assumes that you're running your vegetative grow lights 18 hours per day with just the desk fan, humidifier, heater and manual timer drawing any significant amount of power. In all likelihood, you will not be running your inline fan and carbon filter until the flowering phase, when the plants become more aromatic.

If your base residential rate is around $0.15/ kW, this translates into a monthly expense of approximately $36 for the vegetative phase.

During the flowering phase, which last about 8 weeks you can expect to use your grow lights at maximum power 12 hours per day, your inline fan and carbon filter running 24/7 and the other devices mentioned in the vegetative phase drawing some power as well. This should draw just under 12kW hours per day or 360kW per month. With a base rate of $0.15/ kW, budget $54 per month.

Chapter 6: How Do I Grow a Successful Crop?

I've broken down the growing of your own CBD-rich crops into seven phases. The first phase deals with that all-important step of getting your seeds to germinate. Let's see how you could get this done with minimal frustration and loss.

Phase 1: Germination.

The first order of business once you have your closet grow set up is to source out a reliable source of either cannabis seeds or plants. Then, once we've identified where we're going to obtain our medicinal plants from, then we can look at how to grow healthy seedlings.

Should you be using clones for your starter plants, then most of what is going to be covered in Phase 1 won't apply.

During the germination phase, we want to take your dried out looking seeds, re-hydrate them and plant them in a growing medium once a rootlet (tap root) has pierced the seed's outer shell. This delicate phase can be intimidating for first-time growers, as much of what you'll be experiencing will be a result of trial and error.

To increase your success rate, I'll share one easy-to-follow procedure for germinating your first crop. You may wish to experiment with different approaches down the road. What you're about to learn is a popular, tried and true method.

Types of Cannabis Seeds:

Seeds are available in four different forms, namely:
1. Natural: These seeds are what Mother nature provided, a mixture of female and male plants.
2. Feminized: Developed in India in 1982, all of these seeds produce female plants.
3. Auto-flowering: These plants start to produce flowers within 3 to 4 weeks of germination, no matter what the light regime. You'll see a mixture of males and females.
4. Auto-flowering - Feminized: Plants will auto-flower and all be females.

The least expensive type of seed is the all-natural one. Feminized seeds are costlier than a mixture of natural ones.

Sources of Cannabis Plants:

1. Medical Cannabis Dispensaries:
In jurisdictions where medical cannabis is legal, and where there is a network of cannabis compassion clubs or dispensaries, you may be able to buy seeds locally.

By discretely asking an employee about the possibility of obtaining seeds, you may be able to get a contact number or introduction to a local breeder who has a legal medical garden.

2. Legal Cannabis Seed Stores.
Many countries are moving to legalize the sale of cannabis-related products, including seeds. Depending on your local area, you may be able to find a knowledgeable retailer who can not only provide you with seeds, but also give you some sage advice on how to best cultivate certain strains.

3. Online Seed Banks:
Often Internet cannabis seed re-sellers offer the best selection of seeds to choose from, along with some of the most competitive pricing.

We've been using the same seed bank for years now. Not only do they carry an assortment of popular strains, they're also extensively involved in breeding strains.

4. Local Clone dispensary:
Many states and provinces have well-established cloning facilities that serve the medical marijuana industry. You may be able to obtain clones for your closet grow should you have a doctor-approved medical marijuana prescription. In some jurisdictions, you can purchase a small quantity of clones for personal use to be grown at home.

Selecting a reputable seed bank:

There's nothing worse than the feeling of having been scammed by an online retailer. Not only have you lost some hard-earned cash-ola, you've also lost out in time delays of growing your crop and having to deal with the added stress. Should this happen to you, consider taking some CBD-rich cannabis to help you cope better. May as well walk the talk, right?

To help you avoid being ripped off, here's a 5-step checklist to selecting a reputable seed bank:

1. Professional Online Presence:
As previously mentioned, does the website that you're visiting look like neighbor Bob's 13-year old son built it? Reputable seed companies plan to stick around for the long haul. They're more than likely going to invest in a website that is easy-to-navigate, informative and extensive.

Good online businesses are transparent online. Meaning that they're more than likely to answer a host of frequently asked questions, along with those "should ask" questions potential buyers often pose. They'll also provide multiple means of contacting them should you have questions or concerns.

You may even wish to see if the website URL is registered as a .com or country domain and how long the website has been around by going to Alexa.com or another website for some additional online insights about the seed bank you're investigating.

2. Positive Social Media Reputation:
Are you able to see testimonials coming from 3rd party sources such as Facebook, You Tube or Google? In essence, does the website make a point of providing social proof that they have a positive track record?

You may also be able to find out about the seed bank when visiting forums that discuss topics related to the cannabis industry. Type in "seed bank review forum" in the search bar to see what's currently available. Also, ask around at local cannabis retailers for some possible personal insights into potential seed banks to use.

3. Education:
Does the website have blog posts, dedicated grow pages, or links to articles or videos geared to growing cannabis? Those companies desiring repeat business often go out of their way to educate prospective buyers as to the current best practices for growing cannabis.

4. Multiple Payment Options:
If your only option of paying for the seeds happens to be the newest cryptocurrency, run for the hills. You should be able to access several different payment methods, whether they be by credit card, money order or a payment platform, like PayPal.

5. Shipping Options and Guarantees:
Most seed banks will send you your seeds through the postal system in discreetly packaged bubble envelopes. The seed bank should spell out how your order will be shipped and when to expect your delivery.

Before, you buy any seeds find out via email, web search or a phone call about backorder problems, delivery options, discrete packaging and security arrangements. Most reputable seed banks should be able to get seeds to you within 30 days. Plan your grow accordingly.

And most reputable companies offer some sort of delivery or replacement guarantee should your seeds not arrive or arrive damaged. This has happened to us and the seed bank sent replacement seeds to ensure that we would continue to buy future seeds from them.

Following this checklist, should keep you out of trouble when purchasing seeds online. You may find that some seed banks offer deals on seeds. And, prices for the same variety may vary from seed bank to seed bank. As well, I suggest that you keep accurate records of your grow, especially during the delicate seedling phase. By being proactive, you can more readily demonstrate that you've done everything in your power to optimize your seed propagation should you have a failed grow. Providing a detailed description of your germination process more than likely will result in a positive outcome.

The industry is evolving quickly with new breeders and seed resellers popping up everywhere. Take your time investigating as to which ones hold promise for your particular needs.

What should I buy?

You may wish to begin your search for a cannabis variety suited for your particular ailments or needs by visiting a major cannabis website, such as Leafly.com. This extensive website provides a myriad of information related to some of the most documented and well-known cannabis varieties in the global market. Using the website's search bar, you should be able to identify several strains that could prove beneficial.

A couple of other considerations in your buying decision should be whether or not the variety you would like to grow is suited for an indoor grow and whether or not the variety is easy to grow indoors.

For example, our first CBD-rich cannabis variety was a Harlequin cross from the BC Bud Depot. It was well-suited for a closet grow, being easy to germinate and grow in the confines of a small space.

Seed pricing can vary immensely depending on the type of seed (i.e. natural, feminine, auto-flowering), international reputation (i.e. Cannabis Cup winner) and availability. Expect to pay on average between $5 to $10 per seed.

If you're purchasing natural seeds, buy 10 - 12 seeds since 50% or more may be males once you propagate them. Your male plants will need to be removed from the grow site to prevent them from pollinating your females. If you're planning on spending a little more for feminized seeds, 5 or 6 seeds should be sufficient.

I like to plant 5 or 6 natural seeds when doing a closet grow. This gives me 2 to 4 female plants to work with in my grow tent. More than adequate for my needs. If I'm using feminized seeds, I usually plant 3 at a time since I don't have to worry about culling any males during the flowering phase.

If you're not going to plant all of the seeds at once, store them in a small airtight container placed in a dry, dark, cool place, like your refrigerator. Focus on keeping them dry, so they don't germinate on you inadvertently. Seeds kept dry and cool in the fridge should be viable years down the road.

Seed Germination Timeline:

The germination method that I'm about to share with you involves initially soaking the seeds in water so that they crack, and a tap root emerges. Here's a typical seed germination timeline to help you with your planning:
1. First 24 - 48 hours: Water is absorbed by the seeds and a white root tip cracks the shell casing.
2. First week. Rootlets appear, and the seeds are carefully planted in an initial growing medium. Only watering occurs during the first week.
3. Second week. Root hairs develop in the growing medium and sets of true leaves form. Dilute feeding begins if you're using inert coco coir.
4. Third week. Once three sets of true leaves form, the seedling enters the vegetative growth phase. Dilute feeding begins, if you're using nutrient-rich soil. Should you be using coco coir, continue your feeding regime established in week 2.
5. After 30 days. Any seeds that have not sprouted will in all likelihood not germinate.

What do seedlings like?

Once the seeds have sprouted, the seedlings thrive when certain environmental factors are met, as follows:
1. Light: A light cycle of 18 hours of daylight, followed by 6 hours of complete darkness (18/6 cycle) allows the plants to optimize nutritional uptake and produce healthy roots. Although growers have experimented with 14/10, 16/8 and 24/0 cycles, most growers like to imitate Mother Nature's peak summer daylight schedule. Makes sense, right?

2. Temperature: Seedlings like to grow when the daytime temperature is just below 80°F. Avoid temperature swings of more than 10°F between the evening and day, if you would like to see optimal growth. Wild swings in any of the five environmental factors being described stresses out the plant.

3. Relative Humidity: Keeping the relative humidity of the growing area around 50 - 60% prevents the delicate seedlings from drying out.

4. Ventilation: An exchange of air (carbon dioxide and oxygen) is required for optimal growth. This can be accomplished by opening vents in a domed hot house or using a desk fan set on low to gently circulate the air. Later in the plant's grow cycle, a circulating fan that gently moves your plants will also strengthen the stocks, which will be important for supporting those great big buds during the flowering phase.

5. Nutritional needs: During the various phases of a plant's growth cycle, plants require three essential nutrients in varying percentages. You may have seen the packaging information N-P-K on bottles of nutritional supplements. These are nitrogen, phosphorus and potassium.

Early on, seedlings require higher concentrations of nitrogen to develop strong root structures and develop an expansive leaf canopy. As the flowering phase kicks in, the plants shift to requiring higher concentrations of potassium for bud development.

The important take-away for seedling growth is that very low doses of base nutrients should be administered so as not to chemically burn the delicate seedlings. Each nutritional supplement company will recommend their own feeding regime, and most will recommend that you keep your solution concentration below 300 ppm for the final phase of seedling growth. It's best to err on the side of under-feeding your seedlings during the first two to three weeks of growth, rather than have a major setback should you over-feed. Been there - done it. One particular grow ended up taking a month longer because I fried my little darlings during the seedling phase. Live and learn, right?

6. pH: Controlling pH is essential for stimulating vigorous cannabis plant development. When the pH of your feeding solution is too high (alkaline) or too low (acidic), nutrients cannot be properly absorbed by the plants. By maintaining a nutrient pH level within the range of 5.5 and 6.5, you can assure that your crop has an optimal level of nutrients available. When growing in coco coir, I like to maintain a pH of 6.2 as recommended by the manufacturer. Testing for pH throughout the entire grow operations is essential for producing consistent CBD-rich crops.

Three-step Germination Process:

Step #1: Soaking. Place the number of seeds you would like to germinate in a glass of pH neutral, reverse osmosis/distilled water that's 68°F - 75°F. Soak your seeds anywhere from 12 - 72 hours, until they crack open and a white rootlet begins to appear. They'll probably sink to the bottom of the glass as they hydrate. If you're soaking your seeds for more than 24 hours, replace the water every day. As long as you're replacing the water with clean, oxygenated water, your seeds will not rot. Seeds normally germinate within a few days. And they don't require light in order to do so.

Step #2: Germinating. Once your seeds have developed a rootlet that's about 1/8" long, it's time to remove them from the water. Prepare a damp, unscented paper towel with pH neutral, reverse osmosis/distilled water that's 68°F - 75°F. We want to create a high humidity, warm environment that has some air circulating. To do so, we'll carefully transfer the seeds onto the damp paper towel and fold the towel over, so all sides of the seeds stay moist. Next, we'll place the damp, folded paper towel onto a shallow plate, which we'll keep in a dark environment. Since we do want some air circulation, avoid placing your plate in a small enclosed area like a cupboard or a grow tent.

Be vigilant. Every 6 to 8 hours, check on your seeds to ensure that they are bathed in moisture. Add pH neutral water as needed to keep the paper towels moist, but not overly saturated. I like to spray down the towels. This keeps the towel evenly moist. At no point in time should your paper towels dry out.

Step #3: Transferring. We'll be growing your seedlings in a plastic solo cup or similar container. If you're using an 18-ounce, plastic solo cup, take a pair of scissors and snip three, equally-spaced, water drainage slits in the bottom of the cups, as previously mentioned. Fill each cup 1/2 full, with your growing medium. Why 1/2 full you may be asking? As your seedlings grow, they will stretch up towards your light source. Once they grow just above the lip of each cup, you can carefully add additional growing medium around the delicate stock to provide additional support.

When your seedlings have developed a 1/2" tap root under the paper toweling, it's time to transplant them into your growing medium. Just prior to transplanting, ensure that your growing medium has been watered with reverse osmosis/ distilled water that's been pH'ed down to around 6.2. Water the medium until you're able to collect 10 - 20% of the run-off. You need not add any nutrients during the first week of seedling growth. Each seed has enough food supply for germination.

Now, use a pencil or similar tool to create a 1/4" to 1/2" depth hole in the center of each cup. Carefully transfer each seedling into each individual hole with a pair of clean tweezers or very clean finger tips. Try to place the white rootlet in first. Cover each seedling with a thin layer of growing medium. You want the seed to be totally surrounded by moist medium at a shallow depth.

It's best to place your cups in a climate-controlled environment, like a domed-plastic, hot house. Ideally, you want to create a growing environment that has a relative humidity between 50 - 70%, with a temperature between 70°F - 80°F. If you're using T5 fluorescent lights, position them 2" to 4" above the cups. When your seeds do sprout, you want to have the lights close enough to stimulate growth, yet not so close as to fry your seedlings. To judge if your lights are too close, place hand under the light for 30 seconds at the height of the leaves. Feeling hot? Raise the light slightly.

We have our hot house set up with T5 fluorescent lighting, a seedling heat pad (that came with the hot house), and a 24-hour, manual timer that controls the T5 lighting on an 18-hour on, 6-hour off schedule. We've found that our heating pad tends to be too warm, so we normally place a cardboard or Styrofoam barrier between it and the solo cups. The 18/6 lighting schedule is what we'll be using for our seedling and vegetative growth phases.

We monitor the temperature and humidity with a portable unit that's placed inside the hot house. As needed, we spray down the sides of the dome with clean, neutral water to maintain the humidity above 50%.

Two Alternative Germination Methods:

1. Rock wool cubes:
Rock wool is an inert growing medium that retains moisture and traps air. It is typically sold in sheets of 2" cubes. After your initial glass of water soaking step, place your seeds into pre-soaked rock wool cubes as you would have done with the paper towels. Continue to provide a damp, warm environment during the germination phase.

2. Soil:
In Mother Nature, cannabis seeds fall to the ground during the flowering phase and germinate in the surface soil when conditions are right. Mimicking what naturally occurs in an outdoor growing scenario is an option. You could directly plant your seeds in soil and grow your plants directly in your grow medium. Even though this is nature's way of doing it, you may experience varied results. Not every seed will germinate and grow.

Using Clones?

Most large-scale growers use clones and not seeds as their propagation source. The clones have the same genetic material as the parent and they tend to flower earlier since you're starting with a small plant, rather than seeds.

This may be a viable means of obtaining your plants should you have local access to a small quantity from a dispensary in your jurisdiction. No one currently is shipping clones nationally or internationally. Nor should you risk having clones purchased outside of your home state or province being damaged in transit. Go local and save yourself any headaches.

Locally, clones are typically shipped or transported in small diameter plastic tubes where the clone is inserted into a rockwool plug and then a small amount of water is added before sealing the top. Often the tube will be wrapped in protective bubble wrap before final packaging and shipping or delivery.

Once you receive your clones, handle them with kid gloves, as they will be delicate and in a state of shock due to the shipping ordeal.

Phase 2: Nurturing seedling growth.

You're excited. Your seeds have sprouted. And you see your first pair of immature leaves known as cotyledons growing. Within a few days, your first true set of leaves will appear. Now, it's time to ensure that they thrive in your growing medium. Let's improve the odds of your delicate seedlings surviving the first couple of weeks of development.

This seedling phase typically lasts just a few weeks. You'll enter the vegetative phase when your seedlings have developed three sets of true leaves after the initial cotyledon leaf formation.

Daily Seedling Check-up:

During each of the major growing phases of the plant cycle, you'll be monitoring and adjusting environmental conditions in your closet grow on a daily basis. Sure, it's possible to do so every 2nd day; however, daily observations allow you to react more quickly to problems arising in the seedling hot house or grow tent. I like to check on my babies first thing in the morning, about an hour after the kids wake up when the lights come on.

Here's a daily "to do" list for seedling growth:

1. Record and adjust the temperature and humidity in the grow area.
Opening and closing air vents to regulate air flow and temperature, adjusting any heat pads to provide adequate warmth around 78°F, and refilling room humidifiers are the usual order of business. Your babies need a slight exchange of air, but you also want to avoid any cold drafts hitting them. As well, avoid any unnecessary tampering of your solo cups. The less stress the plants receive, the better the grow.

2. Spray down the dome. The challenge in most grow areas is keeping the relative humidity above 50%, so the seedlings don't dry out too quickly.

3. Assess your plant's reaction to light. If the leaves are curling up, they're open to receiving more light. If down and curled under, they may be telling you that the light source is too close.

4. Look for changes to leaf color. If you're seeing a color change from green to yellow on the tips of the leaves, verify to see if the plants are:
      (i) Receiving too much heat and light.
      (ii) Being overwatered.
      (iii) Suffering from nutrient burn.
      (iv) Drying out at root level.
Once you identify the culprit, adjust accordingly.

5. Water or lightly feed your plants. If your seedling cups weigh significantly less or your moisture meter indicates that the root balls are drying out, then it's time to water. Which brings us to the following question:

When to water and feed?

The answer boils down to two possibilities, whether you're growing in soil or coco coir. When you grow in soil, it contains an adequate supply of essential nutrients for the seedlings to use during the first two weeks of being in the grow medium. Soil requires less intervention. It tends to hold onto water longer than coco coir. You may only need to water your cups every 3rd or 4th day.

On the other hand, coco coir often requires a small amount of watering/ feeding every 2nd day. When using coco coir, you'll need to begin adding a nutrient blend to your watering after the first 7 - 10 days of seedling growth. Being an inert medium, coco coir does not hold onto essential nutrients like soil can. A very dilute nutritional formulation designed for seedling growth is the answer. Count on feeding your seedlings every 4th day. You may occasionally need to water the seedlings with enough water to moisten the roots in between feedings.

One approach to seeing how much water or feed solution to add, is to weight each seedling cup before and after watering. This helps to gauge how much water to use. And how much can you expect to add? I've found that adding 50 - 75 mL (less than 1/4 cup) per solo cup is adequate.

I also like to measure how much water I'm using each time and how much runoff occurs. This gives me a better idea as to how much water is being taken up by the plants. As well, if I'm using a nutrient solution, I'll usually keep the concentration less than 200 to 300 ppm.

Then, I'll measure the runoff with my TDS meter to see if I'm getting an excessive chemical/ nutrient build-up. I'm not too worried if the runoff is less than double the initial concentration level. Your plants only want to take up what they need. However, too strong a nutrient solution becomes toxic to them. When using Diablo nutrients, I use a dilute formulation of Grow, Micro, Bloom and Thrive, along with some Cal-Mag and SM-90.

How could you grow more females from regular seeds?

Each seed has a pre-disposition for one sex over another. Environmental conditions can create hermaphrodites - plants showing characteristics of both sexes. We want to avoid this as much as possible. To do so, here are some simple tips that'll increase the likelihood of your seeds producing more females:

1. Increase the amount of nitrogen during seedling and vegetative growth.
2. Decrease the grow area temperature slightly, keeping it below 78°F.
3. Increase the relative humidity to above 50% during the seedling phase and first part of the vegetative phase.

---

4. Increase the amount of blue spectrum light vs. red. Most LED lighting systems allow you to do this easily.
5. Slightly decrease your plants' exposure to daylight hours from 18 to 16 during the seedling phase and early part of the vegetative phase.
6. Decrease any stress on your plants, especially during transplanting or environmental swings. Make slow changes to your growing environment.

Phase 3: Vegetative Growth.

You're excited again. Your seedlings have developed three true sets of leaves and you're ready to move them into your grow tent, where you can nurture them to produce even more leaf nodes. Let's explore what this short phase has to offer.

Vegetative Phase Goals:

The ultimate goal of the vegetative phase is to create a thick, lush and even canopy of strong cannabis plants, that'll support heavy bud growth during the flowering phase.

This phase normally lasts between 3 to 5 weeks, with 4 weeks being the most common duration when growing CBD-rich strains.

To accomplish this goal, we'll need to:
1. Ensure that an optimal level of nutrients conducive to vegetative and root development is being supplied to the plants.
2. Provide enough light to promote growth.
3. Transplant the seedlings into our final growing pots when an adequate root system has developed along with a sturdy stock.
4. Train each plant to spread out its branches in creating an even, level canopy.

What are the ideal growing conditions during the vegetative phase?

Your plants will thrive best when you place them on an 18:6 light rotation, maintain an air temperature around 78°F with the relative humidity between 50% and 60%, and there is a gentle breeze blowing over your canopy.

You may be tempted to place your lights on a 24-hour cycle. Avoid doing this. Your plants need some dark time to develop both a lush green canopy and strong roots and stock. This only occurs when you allow them to rejuvenate during a short dark period.

Your desk fan serves as your wind source. Direct your breeze over the tops of the canopy or off the sides of your grow tent. You don't want to have the fan blowing directly on the plants, as this causes more negative stress than good when the plants have to be constantly fighting against gale force winds.

Besides your environmental controls, you'll also want to feed your babies with a balanced nitrogen-rich formulation. As the plants grow, the amount of nutrients added to each feeding formulation will also grow. You may start with a solution concentration around 500 ppm and end up after 4 weeks of vegetative growth with a solution concentration around 800 ppm. This seems to be the sweet spot for many cannabis grows. Any higher and you risk chemically burning your plants. Any lower and your plants may show signs of slow growth or yellowing of the leaves.

Daily Vegetative Check-up:

Just as we've done for the seedling phase, we're going to monitor our closet grow on a regular basis. Here's a daily "to do" list for vegetative growth:

1. Record and adjust the temperature and humidity in the grow tent. You may need to open and close air vents, adjust your space heater or refill your tent humidifier in order to properly adjust your temperature and humidity.

2. Assess each plant's uptake of fluids. Lift each pot to see how dry it may be getting. If the pot seems 50% lighter, it probably requires watering. Should you have a soil moisture meter, verify how dry your root ball is becoming.

3. Assess your plant's reaction to light. As in the seedling daily checklist, look at your plants' leaves for signs of over or under-stimulation. Adjust your canopy height from the LED light source by using the racket system that you've set up with the lights.

4. Water or lightly feed your plants. Consider watering/feeding your plants at the beginning of the lights-on schedule to increase uptake. Also, ensure that you vigorously shake each bottle before use to thoroughly mix the chemicals together. For greater accuracy, I like to use a small, 3-cc. plastic syringe. I pour a small amount of nutrient solution into a shot glass. Then, I draw up just the right amount of solution into my syringe. I discard any excess solution left in the shot glass, rather than risking cross contamination of my bottles. It's important to get into the practice of establishing good feeding habits so that you don't run into problems down the road. Also, water in a circular motion around the periphery of your container. Roots grow out from the center. Water so that they don't dry out.

A typical feed/water rotation cycle to consider using for coco coir is to:
> (i) Feed - Day 1.
> (ii) Dry - Day 2.
> (iii) Light Water - Day 3.
> (iv) Dry - Day 4.
> (v) Feed - Day 5. repeating the cycle.

When using coco coir, you'll find that the top 1/2" of coconut fibers will be dry to the touch prior to the next watering/feeding. This is normal. What is not normal is having that dry layer extend an inch or more down into the pot. As a simple rule of thumb that you can modify for your particular growing conditions, consider using up to 2 gallons (8 L) of solution for a 2' x 4' grow with new plants.

After watering your plants, test the TDS level (concentration) of the runoff. When you allow your plants to dry down too much, salts are left behind in the medium. Should you feed your plants the next time, the combined combination may be too much for the plants. This is why you should follow a feed/water cycle described above. It does a gentle flush of the growing medium.

Use a small shop vacuum, turkey baster or large syringe to remove any excess runoff. In a pinch you could mop it up with an old towel.

During this phase I normally don't bother trying to measure the quantity of runoff as it disturbs the grow too much.

If you're interested in augmenting vegetative growth during this growth phase, you could install a portable CO_2 - enhancer that'll emit a steady stream of CO_2 into the grow tent. Or, you could do what I've often done, place glass carboys of fermenting beer or wine by the closet grow. Yes, I'm also an accomplished brewer of all-grain, hand-crafted ales.

How to transplant seedlings:

At some point during the vegetative phase, you'll be transplanting your seedlings from their individual cups into larger pots. I like to do this about one week after the seedlings have been introduced to the grow tent, since I use a hot house for seedling growth. The delicate seedlings need a short period of time to acclimate to their new surroundings.

During that week of acclimation, I'll slowly lower my LED lights from 32" to 24", which is what is recommended with the lighting system that I'm using. You'll need to see what your particular system recommends. I'm also making small adjustments to the ventilation, humidity and temperature so that these parameters fall within my ideal range.

At week's end, I'll prepare my pots. I like to use 5-gallon Smart pots filled with rinsed coco coir medium. I prefer not having to do more than one transplant per entire grow cycle. The less hands-on work I do, the better it is for the plants.

The coco coir is rinsed with reverse osmosis water that has been pH'ed down to about 6.2. I usually time my transplant to coincide with a feeding. So, I also prepare an appropriate feeding solution. But I also add a few drops of TanLin to the feed. This decrease the odds of having any bugs being introduced into the closet grow.

To prep my Smart pots, I start by filling the bottom 1/2 of each pot with coco coir growing medium. Then, I place the same-sized, solo cup in the medium as my seedling cups. I pack my rinsed coco coir around it. By carefully removing the cup, you'll end up with a perfect hole for transplanting your individual seedlings. Your hole will be exactly the same size as the solo cup you're using.

If you have mycorrhizae, now's the time to place a small amount according to the directions and spreading it in the hole you've created in your pot. Lightly moisten the mycorrhizae with a fine spray of clean water.

Removing the seedling from my solo cup is easy. I'll wet the coco coir medium with reverse osmosis water pH'ed to 6.2 so that the plug I'm removing retains most of its shape. I position myself over my pot and place my hand over the top of the container, gently cradling the plant's stem between my fingers. Then, I slowly turn the cup upside down and allow the plug to slip out while guiding it into the hole. I gently press my plug into place to remove any air gaps. Finally, I water with my nutrient solution and remove any run-off from my drip tray. Piece of cake, right?

Why do so many grows result in failure?

Most novice growers who experience a crop failure or less than optimal bud development report that it's due to five common errors, namely:
1. Over-watering. This is a hard one to correct, if you don't know how much is enough. I've shared some insights into how much you could be using, along with ways of determining if you're under or over-watering your babies. Over-watering drowns the roots, deprives them of oxygen and makes them susceptible to fungal attack. Over-watering will show up in slow plant growth, leaves that curl down and yellow, soggy soil and fungal growth.

To avoid this problem, ensure that your plants are receiving adequate ventilation during the growing phase. As well, make sure that you draw off any run-off, so the roots don't sit in a pool of stagnant water.

2. Over-feeding. Medical cannabis growers often kill their plants with too much kindness in providing too much nutrition or too much of one nutrient. By using a "complete" nutritional system and following the company's recommendations, you're more than likely to stay out of trouble. Most combi-pack solution sets sold by cannabis nutrient companies will do the trick. If you're using a nutritional system designed for plants and vegetables in general, err on the side of caution by reducing the concentration of each feed until you know if the formulation is becoming too toxic for your plants.

3. Too much light intensity. If some light is good, more should be better, right? There's a fine line between optimizing your light intensity for a grow and causing leaf damage. Be careful not to fry branches of your plants. This can occur if you're not training your plants to spread out and create an even canopy. We'll get into that in a moment. Follow your light manufacturer's suggestions as to what the distance should be between the light source and your canopy.

4. Improper air flow. If you're not ventilating and exchanging stale air in your tent and replacing it with fresh air you run the risk of creating some big headaches. Without air flow mold and mildew will take hold. Without air exchange your plants won't be able to transpire properly. A fresh supply of oxygen and carbon dioxide is required for optimal plant growth. Keep your desk fan running 24/7 and have ventilation spots open in the upper section of your grow tent to encourage proper air flow.

5. Bug infestations. If you've embraced my pro-active approach to dealing with those nasty little plant eaters, then you should be able to control your grow environment quite well. A combination of physical traps and chemical deterrents works best. Should an infestation take hold, check with a local horticulturalist for chemical treatments you could use that won't create toxic buds in the end.

What is canopy management?

Canopy management is crucial to being able to optimize your bud yield. The goal of following some sort of canopy management system is to create an even canopy with bud-producing branches (colas) covering the entire tent footprint so that you can get the maximum amount of bud from your plants.

And how will we achieve this goal? By creating a screen of green or what is known as a SCRoG. Did I mention that you needed to invest in some nylon netting? Well, this is where we'll be putting it to good use.

We won't be setting up our SCRoG net until the beginning of the flowering phase. However, it's important to understand why we're doing certain things in preparation for flowering. When we change the light cycle during the flowering phase, the plants will develop sexually. And once we know which plants are male or female, we'll remove the males and work with the remaining females in setting up the SCRoG.

As well, we'll introduce a few canopy management techniques that'll start training our plants to develop a flat even canopy. During most of the vegetative phase, your kids will remain undisturbed, receiving some nutrition and water to foster growth.

Why SCRoG?

Since we are in a restrictive space - a closet. And, you're more than likely using a grow tent that has a maximum height of 5'. We need to plan out our vertical grow space very carefully, so as not to have our light source so close to our buds that it damages them or reduces the quality of the CDB-rich resin we so desire.

This is where the technique of SCRoGing comes in. By setting up a screen we can train our plants to spread out over the entire footprint of the tent. We'll do this by bending and weaving branches through the holes in the screen. This means that we can set the height of our canopy so that we're able to use the optimal light intensity of our LED lighting system.

151

Here's how a typical closet tent grow shakes out. For example, a 5-gallon Smart pot should have a maximum height of just under 12". You'll allow your plants to grow vertically about 8" to 10" before setting up your SCRoG netting. This distance allows you to still water and prune (trim) your plants. As your plants grow during the flowering phase, they'll extend up through the netting. However, because you've been training them, your canopy will be at an even height. In most cases, your canopy can grow comfortably another foot before being too close to your light source.

You'll need about 8" of headspace at the top of your grow tent for setting up your inline fan system and lighting. Most LED light systems recommend an 18" space between the canopy and lights during the final weeks of the flowering phase. This is the distance where optimal growth occurs. By SCRoGing, we're able to get the most out of both our plants and lighting, while still being confined to a space the size of a closet.

To summarize, here's what a cross section of your grow tent will look like during the flowering phase:
1. Your pot will rise up to about 12" in height.
2. The SCRoG net will be positioned 8" - 10" above the level of the soil.
3. The top of your canopy will grow to a height of 12" above the SCRoG.
4. Your lighting will be positioned 18" to 20" above the canopy.
5. Your air filtration system along with the lights will occupy 8" to 10" of headspace at the top of your 5' tent.

How do I prepare my plants for my SCRoG net?

The two main techniques that we'll use in conjunction with the SCRoG net are:
1. Topping.
2. Low stress training.

Let's take a look at each of these to see how each technique helps us achieve our ultimate goal of an evenly-spaced, flat canopy.

1. Topping. The first technique to use during the 3rd or possibly 4th week of your vegetative cycle involves removing a newly formed leaf site at the top of your plant to encourage branching. Instead of one pair of leaves forming, two pairs will be created. This increases the number of bud sites available as the plant grows. It also makes the training of your plant easier down the road.

Topping occurs after your pants have formed 5 true sets of leaves, with the 5th set of leaves being 1/4" to 1/2" long. And it should be done no later than one week before switching to flowering. This normally means that with a 4-week veg cycle, you'll want to top your plants during the 3rd week.

The procedure is a simple one. Just squeeze the base of your 5th node and gently pluck the node, small leaves and all from the stem. Should you screw things up and fail to remove the entire bud, the resulting topping is called a FIM (F***k, I Missed), which is perfectly okay.

Topping will result in creating a 4-way plant with 4 symmetrical arms. Which brings us to training those newly formed branches.

2. Low stress training. Once your new branches develop, you'll tie down each arm of your 4-way plant using a low stress training method. Start shaping all four arms so that they grow horizontally by using gentle, even, downward pressure. Keep even pressure on the arms, so that the main stem is not pulled in one direction. Then use a safety pin and twist tie to attach each arm to your pot during training. Avoid using thin, razor-sharp ties like wire, fishing line or dental floss to hold down the branches.

You could repeat the topping process once again, but this is not necessary under normal growing situations. Should you decide to do a 2nd topping, allow your babies to grow out 2 to 5 days, before doing it. You'll also want to extend your veg cycle by 5 to 7 days, as well.

Other than using these two canopy management techniques, you'll have minimal direct contact with your plants. You're now well on your way to producing a lush green canopy from which your CBD-rich buds will sprout.

Phase 4: Flowering.

You're excited even more because this is where all the action occurs. Your bushy little plants are ready to enter their sexual development phase, where you'll be able to nurture your females and vote your males off the island. The flowering phase involves several aspects, namely:

1. Sexing the plants and culling the males.
2. Using SCRoGing to encourage bud development across an even canopy that'll occupy your entire tent footprint.
3. Flushing excess chemicals/ nutrients from your plants during the final week of flowering.

Flowering Phase Goals:

The primary goal of the flowering phase is to develop multiple bud sites, coated with CBD-rich resin devoid of any chemical residues and ready for harvest at the peak of their resin production. Boy ...that was like spitting out a mouthful of clams!

During the flowering phase, cannabis flowers grow and pack together to form dense nuggets called colas. This is what we'll be harvesting after they achieve optimal ripeness.

The flowering phase normally lasts 8 weeks when growing CBD-rich strains indoors.

To accomplish this goal, we'll need to:

1. Ensure that an optimal level of nutrients conducive to bud development is being supplied to the plants. This means slowly switching from a nitrogen-rich feeding formulation to one rich in potassium.
2. Change the light cycle to promote bud growth, rather than vegetative growth. Switching your lights from an 18:6 to a 12:12 cycle will cause sexual development of your plants.
3. Identify male plants early in the flowering phase and vote them off Survivor (remove them).
4. Continue to train each plant to spread out its branches in creating an even, level canopy using our SCRoG netting.
5. Managing the underside of the canopy so that non-productive shoots and leaves are removed.

What are the ideal growing conditions during the flowering phase?

Your plants will thrive best when you place them on an 12:12 light rotation, maintain an air temperature around 78°F with the relative humidity dropping from 50+% to under 40% by the end of flowering. In nature, as cannabis plants detect changes in the environment that fall is approaching, the plant goes into "survival of the species" mode. To ensure continued survival of the plant species for generations to come, they develop sexually and if given the opportunity, they'll propagate, developing seeds in the process.

As well, about mid-way through your flowering phase, you'll probably fire up your inline fan and carbon filter as the sweet smell of cannabis begins to waif through your closet. Continue to direct the breeze created by your desk fan over the tops of the canopy or off the sides of your grow tent. Remember to avoid having the fan blowing directly on the plants, which'll cause them to struggle.

Your light intensity will kick up a notch as you switch from blue spectrum light to full spectrum blue/red light. This concentrated 12-hour exposure to a higher light intensity will cause a dramatic shift in bud site development.

Do you remember what determines the maximum yield you can expect from your grow op?

Here are those factors in the context of your flowering phase:
1. Amount of light (distance) and type of light (spectrum). Your LED lights will not only switch to a more intense, fuller light spectrum, but you'll also position them closer to the canopy to optimize growth.
2. Size of the canopy (tent dimensions). Your SCRoGing will produce an even, flat canopy where bud sites can grow at the same rate.
3. Light penetration through the canopy. You'll be pruning the canopy so that extraneous, underdeveloped or drying leaves are removed to expose healthy, productive leaves.

4. Proper watering and feeding (nutrition). You'll continue to feed and water your plants, slowly switching from a nitrogen-rich formulation to a potassium-rich one.
5. Maintain an ideal temperature and humidity range. You'll foster bud development by slowly manipulating the growing environment so that it becomes less humid and cooler over time, as in nature in many areas of the world.

Daily Flowering Check-up:

As with the vegetative growth check-up, you'll follow the same steps along with a couple of extras:

1. Record and adjust the temperature and humidity in the grow tent. Open and close air vents. Adjust your space heater. And refill your tent humidifier in order to control your grow environment. (We often remove the humidifier and heater mid-way through flowering in order to reduce both the temperature and humidity).

2. Monitor any odors coming from your closet grow. Turn on your inline fan and decrease the fan speed with the fan controller once a faint odor arises. Once you have your fan going, close all top vents, leaving only one or two small bottom vents open to draw fresh air into the bottom of your tent.

3. Assess each plant's uptake of fluids. You probably won't want to lift each pot to see how dry it may be getting, since this may disturb your SCRoGing. Should you have a soil moisture meter, verify how dry your root ball is becoming with the meter.

4. Assess your plant's reaction to light. Look at your plants' leaves for signs of over or under-stimulation. Adjust your canopy height from the LED light source by using the racket system set up with the lights. Remember, we're increasing both the intensity and spectrum of light being made available to your flowering plants.

5. Feed and water your plants - according to the cycle you've set up during the vegetative phase. As the plants grow, the amount of nutrients added to each feed with increase. Most feeding regimes will have you start around 800 ppm and end up after 6 weeks of flower growth with a solution concentration around 1000 to 1200 ppm. As a rule of thumb, consider using 3.0 to 4.5 gallons (11 - 17L) of solution for a well-established grow in a 2' x 4' tent. Also, try to maintain a solution temperature in the range of 70°F to 75°F.

6. Look for signs of sexual development - during the first two weeks of flowering. The goal is to have unpollinated female plants develop without any seed production. This is called "sinsemilla" development.

How do you tell the sexes apart?

As so aptly put by a 5-year old in the movie Kindergarten Cop with Arnold Schwarzenegger who was intently looking on: "Boys have penises and girls have vaginas." Yes, you will be lifting up leaves and looking for sexual changes in your plants every day in the early stages of the flowering phase.

You'll be looking for specific changes in the upper nodes of your plants where sexing typically occurs first. Since males tend to show signs of sexual development first, it's often easier to identify them early during flowering and remove them before they release any pollen. Be vigilant the last week of the grow cycle, just in case your males decide to show off their manliness early.

Male plants are usually taller than female plants. They tend to have stout stems, sporadic branching and fewer leaves. This is because in Mother Nature gravity and wind carry male pollen down from above to land on any females below. The top regions of your plants are where to start looking for pre-flowers. Pre-flowers often emerge at the 4th or 5th node where the emerging branch meets the stock. This area is known as the stipule. It is at this junction that the sex organs or calyx will develop.

157

Males flowers develop a calyx that often looks like a ball hanging off a small, short stem (stamen). Whereas, female pre-flowers tend to be nestled into the stipule and have a more tapered appearance with the formation of a pair of fine white hairs (pistils).

For a more detailed look at the differences, check out You Tube postings using the search term "how to sex cannabis plants".

If your grow has been a stressful one, look for signs of plants that develop both sets of sex organs becoming hermaphrodite plants. Remove these plants from your grow tent along with any males as soon as possible.

Setting up your SCRoG:

Once you've removed any suspicious culprits, it's time to set up your SCRoG net in your tent and begin training those little darlings. I have my nylon net stretched over and attached to a 2' x 4' PVC pipe frame with nylon cable ties. This allows me to easily move the entire frame up and down in the tent. And since the elbow joints aren't glued in place, the whole assembly quickly comes apart for easy storage. You could also directly attach your netting to the four inner poles of your grow tent eliminating the frame altogether. However, the frame does offer more support and control over how your canopy evolves.

At what height should you set up your netting? Being in a closet, vertical space is at a premium. So, we want to create a low-lying canopy that allows our LED lighting system to function at an optimal level without damaging your crop. Try to maintain a distance of 8" to 10" above the level of your soil with your net. You want to keep things compact. However, you still want to be able to feed your babies and occasionally trim underneath your canopy.

So far, you've sent your male plants packing home, you have your SCRoG net set up and now you're wondering what to do next, am I right? The answer is - canopy management.

Canopy Management:

The two techniques you'll be using to create that ideal canopy are:
1. Low stress training within the netting.

2. Pruning to eliminate extraneous or counter-productive foliage.

1. Low stress training. As your plant colas (branches) grow up through the netting, gently tuck them under the netting once they're 2" to 3" above it. Bend only those branches that are supple enough to avoid injury (to the plant, not you silly). Eventually, you'll weave the colas up and down through the netting, moving them to every nook and cranny of your tent. Move each cola only one square's distance at a time. You may find that as your plants grow, you'll need to move certain branches over. The ultimate goal is to create a 6" to 8" thick even canopy above the netting during the final stages of flowering.

2. Pruning. Although pruning (trimming shoots and leaves) is Verboten during the veg phase, we'll be using it to create a thick layer of foliage, whereby all of the leaves are impacted by your LED lighting and contribute to overall plant growth. Pruning also improves air flow around your plants, as well as helps to decrease the humidity levels in your grow tent during the final stages of the flowering phase.

Pruning does not remove strong, healthy leaves. In essence, pruning removes dead leaves, underdeveloped shoots and growth that hinders optimal plant development. The latter happens when the plant develops branches that don't receive much of the light of day and are beginning to yellow.

When pruning, err on the side of caution by going slowly. Take your time removing extraneous growth from the plant. Removing more than 20% of the foliage in a short time span will result in excessive stress and poorer bud development.

As well, always use clean tools when pruning. Wiping down your instruments with rubbing alcohol or a mild bleach solution will kill most microbes.

Now, that your plants are trained, well-fed and growing like weeds. Heck! They are weeds. It's time to look at reducing the amount of chemical buildup in your plants. This is known as flushing.

Although there is some controversary as to the efficacy of this technique, most commercial growers flush their crops, despite a lack of peer-reviewed scientific research that would support such a practice.

How do you flush your plants?

No toilet bowls required for this operation. During week seven of the flowering phase and approximately one week before harvesting your crop, you'll thoroughly water your cannabis plants with clean water. Shoot for a temperature around 75°F with a pH of 5.8 to 6.0. These conditions are conducive to dissolving nutrients held in your grow medium.

Flushing removes any chemical built up in your growing medium but does not remove any appreciable amount being stored in the plant itself. This forces the plants to use the balance of the nutrients in their system before harvest. To do so, flush your plants at least 5 to 6 days before harvesting.

You'll require about 1 gallon of water for each gallon of soil - five gallons of water for a 5-gallon Smart pot. What I like to do is set a 20-minute time and water my plants within that time frame. Doing so, ensures that I'm not over-watering and causing more harm than good. As you water your plants, remove any excess water with a shop vac or other means. I've even used a submersible aquarium pump in a pinch.

After flushing, you won't be adding any nutrients back into the soil, just a final watering about 2 days before harvesting. And when should you harvest? We'll look at the optimal time to do so in the following phase.

Phase 5: Harvesting.

You're rubbing your hands together like a giddy child in anticipation of getting a candy treat, waiting impatiently to harvest those resin-coated nuggets that are crying out to you. During the last couple of weeks of the flowering phase, we want to assess how the resin is forming on your buds.

During bud development, the stigmas, which are fuzzy, pollen-catching pistil hairs on your buds, will be white in color. They are used in reproductive growth and do not contain any CBD-rich resin.

What you're looking for are the resin-coated bulbous glands (trichomes) that are found on the buds. Under a magnifying lens, these glands initially look like clear or translucent stocks with large shiny bulbous heads. As your buds reach ripeness, they'll swell with resin and the trichomes will become more prominent and erect.

When should you harvest your crop?

A cannabis plant's flowering cycle, along with its ripening and harvesting time, are variety specific. Most indoor grows harvest during the 8th week of the flowering phase at the tail end of flushing. To determine the optimal time to harvest does require a bit of experience. However, we can use two parameters to help us in our decision-making process, namely:
1. Pistil Coloration: When those tiny white hairs become 50% to 70% brown in color, you'll generally produce a bud that is lighter in taste. At 70% to 90% coloration, peak taste will be reached.

2. Trichome Coloration: Look for an abundance of milky white trichomes. Too much amber color? Harvest right away. The glands are starting to rupture, and the resin is beginning to volatize into the air, resulting in few potent cannabinoids being left behind.

To get a sense of what everything looks like from a microscopic point of view pop on over to You Tube and search for "when to harvest cannabis".

What do you need to get ready?

During the last week of ripening, inspect your buds on a daily basis to assess how the pistils and trichomes appear. You could also trim fan leaves found at the bottom of your plants that aren't getting light or that are blocking buds from receiving direct light.

Consider partially de-leafing your plants the night before harvesting. Look at de-leafing as being the removal of up to half of the under-canopy just prior to harvesting, thus possibly reducing some trimming and drying time later.

Once you've established a harvest date, prepare the tools and supplies you'll need beforehand. Stop watering your plants 2 to 3 days beforehand. And consider placing your plants in a 24-hour period of darkness the day before harvesting. It's best to harvest just after your plants have gone through a full dark cycle. Cannabinoids accumulate more during this period of time.

Also, decreasing the air temperature of your indoor grow environment to 65°F - 68°F with a relative humidity just below 50%, helps retain volatile terpenes from evaporating and reduces the incidence of mold occurring.

Set up your work station with a comfortable chair or stool, large catch basin (or spare drip tray), rubbing alcohol for cleaning your tools, pruning snips/ sheers, surgical gloves, plastic bags for your resin-coated trim leaves, paper towels and a measuring scale.

After you harvest your plants, you'll quickly wipe down your grow tent with a dilute solution of hydrogen peroxide or bleach and set it up for the drying phase. We want to eliminate the chances of any mold or fungus spores infesting the drying area.

Any resin-coated trim leaves close to your buds can be placed in the plastic bag suitable for the freezer. The bag can then be placed in the freezer for future processing. We double bag our leaves so as to reduce the smell of cannabis emanating from the freezer. You'll want to remove as many of the resin-coated trichomes on these leaves to produce a product called kief. When you separate the resin-rich trichomes from plant material you end up with a yellow or pale green powder called kief. Recall that kief can then be used to create edibles, tinctures and oils, which you'll learn about at the end of this section.

Growers have three ways of harvesting their crops:
1. **Whole plant**. Buds are processed all at once, whether they're all ripe or not. Drying of the whole plant once suspended, is a slower more even drying process. The biggest disadvantage is that it takes up more room, and space is at a premium in a closet grow.

2. *Branches*. Cutting branches is often more convenient than dealing with the whole plant. You'll spend a bit more time doing so; however, the resulting material is easier to handle in a small space.

3. *Whole ripe buds*. Wet trimming buds requires more time up front. The biggest advantage is that you'll end up with less material to have to dry.

Although you could harvest your buds each day as they reach optimal ripeness over the course of a week, this approach may not be pragmatic for a discrete, closet grow. I prefer harvesting on a specific day, as do most closet growers.

Trimming is the process of separating the highest quality parts of the plant from the stems and leaves, which we'll dispose of or compost. What we desire are the CBD-rich buds and any sugar leaves that grow next to the buds. Those "sugar-coated" leaves located right next to the buds contain resin that has fallen onto them. This is a rich source of cannabinoids that we can separate and process later as kief.

Since I have a portable, nylon, drying rack that I suspend in my grow tent, I tend to wet trim my buds on harvest day. Recall that wet trimming is the process of removing buds and leaves from the plant on harvest day, leaving you with less work to do once they're dry. Wet trimmed buds are then dried on trays or screens, which take up less space in your tent. You'll also find that the total drying phase is shorter by processing your buds all at once with this approach.

Dry trimming is the removal of buds and leaves from the plant or branches after the drying phase. Most closet growers opt for doing a branch harvest and dry trimming once the buds have reached an optimal level of dryness. The dry buds are easier to cut and handle. This process is described below.

Your goal when branch trimming is to cut branches from each plant that are approximately the same length so that they all dry evenly at roughly the same time. Try to cut the stalks at a 90° right angle. Cutting at a 45° angle results in one sharp, poke your eye out for sure, hazard.

We'll suspend these branches from either plastic hangers or drape them over a rope once we've emptied the grow tent of its pots, lights and humidifier. All that you'll need during the drying phase is your desk fan and carbon filter with the inline fan set up.

Let's take a look at the drying and curing phase in more detail.

Phase 6: Drying & Curing.

The main goal of the drying and curing phase of your closet grow is to produce both CBD-rich bud and sugar-coated leaves that can either be stored long-term or further processed to produce edibles, tinctures, ointments and oils.

Drying should be done slowly in a dark, cool environment in order to preserve terpenes and flavonoids that give the buds their distinctive aroma, flavor and benefits.

To avoid fungus or bacterial problems, try keeping the temperature of your grow tent cool between 62°F and 68°F with the relative humidity between 40% and 50%. Having your desk fan blowing off the sides of your grow tent with the inline fan running, will remove moist air and odors from the tent.

When is drying complete?

As you observe the drying process unfolding over the course of several days, you'll notice that the buds will lose their green color and water weight. They'll begin to turn shades of yellow, brown, red and purple while becoming denser and brittle looking.

Your buds will begin to feel dry on the outside while still being pliable on the inside with some moisture being retained. Gently take a medium-sized bud in your hands (after you've washed your hands of course) and slowly bend the bud in half. If the bud stem bends, it's still too damp. If it breaks or snaps, your buds are ready for dry trimming and curing.

Another technique is to take one of your branches, locate a side stem that contains a bud and try to snap the bottom end. If it makes a subtle snapping noise, as opposed to just bending, it's ready to cure.

A rough guideline for drying times using the branch method under the ideal environmental conditions described is 5 to 7 days.

Should you have large nuggets from the cannabis variety that you're growing, consider allowing these buds to dry a little bit longer. Being larger and denser, they may require more time for the moisture to escape the core and not end up being moldy.

Although you may be tempted to use a "quick dry" method to processing your bud, be advised that most of these methods result in a minty chlorophyll taste and a harsher smoke/ vape.

How do I hand trim my dry buds?

Here's a six-step process to follow:
1. Starting with clean, gloved hands remove a foot-long section of branching to process.
2. Trim and discard any extraneous material (stalks and fan leaves), not near any buds.
3. Remove any sugar leaves found right next to each bud and place them in a plastic container or bag for later processing.
4. Once any curled-up sugar leaves have been removed from the buds, clip each bud from the cola or branch. Keep your bud size under 3" in length so that they will cure properly after the drying phase.
5. Set both the dried buds and sugar leaves aside for weighing. This is where it gets exciting; seeing what quantity of CBD-rich medicine you've grown over the course of the past 4 months.
6. After weighing your buds, loosely place them in glass containers (mason jars used for canning work well) that are up to 3/4 full. Air space is important as you will see.

Now, we're ready to "burp" our babies over the course of the next few weeks.

What is burping?

Burping is the systematic exchange of ambient air with air that's enclosed in your jars. This is part of the curing process, whereby you're transforming "green" bud into a pleasant final product that can be enjoyed for months to come. Like most red wines, your buds will improve over time as they cure and age. Of note is that curing does not make buds more potent than they already are. Well-cured buds produce a smooth, flavorful taste.

Here's a simple process:
1. Place your partially filled and sealed jars in a cool, dark area, such as your grow tent.
2. Wait 4 - 6 hours. Look to see if your buds are sweating. Sweating indicates that they are too wet and need to dry more. Open the jars for several minutes (burp the jar) to release excess moisture.
3. Wait another 12 hours. Repeat the burping process. Later the 2nd day, repeat the burping looking for any condensation. The ideal relative humidity level that you're trying to achieve is between 55% and 62%. Daily air exchange is crucial to reducing the chances of any anaerobic bacteria setting up and ruining your harvest.
4. For the remaining 5 days of the week, burp your buds every 24 hours (more so if needed). For each burping during the first week, carefully remove and re-arrange the buds in each jar.
5. After the first week, you can switch to burping your bud every other day. Open up the jars for one minute before re-sealing them. Continue to do so for at least another week.
6. At a minimum, cure your bud for 14 days before smoking or vaping the product if you're looking for a tasty experience. Then, get into the habit of inspecting your bud on a weekly basis thereafter. When pinched, a nug should be dry on the surface, but should bounce back from squeezing much like a sponge.

Phase 7: Optimal Storage.

Once buds are dried and cured, they are at their peak for potency. Marijuana loses its potency over time. For example, over a 2-year period of storage at room temperature THC gradually degrades by 25% to CBN, which is less psychoactive. Hence, the rationale for producing your medicine on a regular basis, preferably twice a year. This may be more important when growing varietals that contain a higher percentage of THC, as opposed to cultivars that are almost entirely CBD.

Storing buds in a freezer or refrigerator slows deterioration. A freezer is best for long-term storage over a year long. A refrigerator works well for preserving your buds when consumed within the year.

Buds stored in the freezer long-term must be dried properly to prevent unnecessary condensation and freezer burn. They should also be handled delicately as the resin-coated glands become brittle and easily shaken off.

Storage at room temperature is also an option. A cool, dry, dark environment works best for preserving the freshness of your bud. Shoot for temperatures below 68°F to preserve the terpene profile.

Light, especially UV light, will quickly erode the quality of your buds. For this reason, try to use opaque glass jars or coffee canisters, unless you'll be storing your containers in a completely dark environment.

Glass makes a great, inert, solid storage container as it won't pick up odors. Clear glass is your cheapest option with violet glass being the most expensive one. Violet glass blocks visible light with the exception of violet light. Clear glass must be kept out of any light, while violet glass can be kept out in the open.

Another storage alternative is stainless steel. These airtight, lightweight containers block out 100% of the light. They usually come with a locking mechanism that makes them airtight. However, their initial cost can be a deterrent in purchasing them.

Plastic containers are one option to consider, but as a last resort, since the slightly acidic buds degrade certain plastics. We like to use a vacuum, coffee canister for short-term storage of our buds. Any bud stored in our coffee canister is used up within a couple of months.

There are other methods to store bud that you may wish to explore at some later time these include vacuum-sealing and gas-based sealing.

How could I test my cannabis for cannabidiol levels?

At some point, you may be asking yourself how do I determine what percentage of cannabinoids my recent harvest contains? There are two ways to proceed, namely:
1. Do-It-Yourself Test Kits.
2. Bio-Technical Testing Labs.

The most cost-effective way to test for approximate levels of CBD and THC is to pick up a do-it-yourself test kit designed for the cannabis industry. We like to use the kits from Compassionate Analytics CBD / THC test kits. They are one of the least expensive options out in the market.

The kits come in two forms, one to test CBD and another for testing THC levels. For about $50 per kit, you'll have enough in your testing kit to do 5 tests. The testing procedure is easy and accurate enough for a home grow environment. You can test your variety in under 10 minutes for less than $10 per test using their colorimetric strip technology. In essence, you'll match the color of your treated sample with a color grid that corresponds to a specific cannabinoid concentration level. Each kit contains the analytical tools you require for quick and accurate testing of either CBD or THC.

Bio-technical testing labs can be found with a quick Internet search. There are more than 50 in The United States. Canada has more than a dozen laboratories authorized to provide testing services to individuals who would like a simple potency testing done. For example, a basic potency test in Canada by Supra THC Services will run you about $75 CAD, while one in the United States will cost you about $50 US per basic test.

Testing of your cannabis is not a "have to" decision. But it sure helps. By testing for potency, you're now armed with some basic information as to how to better control dosing when you're making edibles, tinctures, oils and ointments.

Let's take a look at post-harvest production in our final phase of cannabis production - Making CBD-Rich Products.

Chapter 7. How Do I Produce My Own Medicinal Products?

This stand-alone chapter addresses the question of how you could make a variety of CBD-rich products that are currently available commercially in the retail market. Making your own medicinal products opens up a myriad of therapeutic possibilities for the cannabis that you choose to grow. Not only this, you'll also save a ton of money not having to pay retail for the products that you do produce at home.

Phase 8: Making CBD-Rich Products.

After your harvest, you'll end up with two grades of product:
1. CBD-rich buds.
2. Resin-coated sugar leaves (also known as shake).

The buds can be used for smoking or better yet - vaping. A portion can also be used to produce kief, which will be the base ingredient that we'll use for creating all sorts of other products. We like to set aside any immature buds with our sugar leaves for this purpose. As for the sugar leaves or shake, we'll need to separate the organic material from the resinous glands before we can use it in a variety of products.

Depending on what tickles your fancy, there is a cost associated with creating these products. Factor this into your overall budget based on what method of processing you believe will be the most beneficial to you or your loved ones.

Which brings us to ... how to make kief using a simple extraction method that uses water, ice and agitation followed by filtering. You'll end up producing a somewhat compact, wet kief known as water hash. This water hash will serve as your base ingredient in making an assortment of high-quality products.

Sure, you could use dried buds or shake to make many of these products. However, by starting with kief or water hash as a concentrate, you'll end up with products that taste better (no green, minty flavors to put up with - unless you're crazy like me and like that sort of thing). Not to mention that any edible products being produced are easier to digest when using a kief-based concentrate.

How to make water hash:

I'll describe a couple of ways of making water hash, depending on whether or not you would like to invest in micron filtration bags or not. Given the choice, the 1st method, which uses Bubble Bags is the way to go if you want to produce an optimal amount of quality kief from your buds and trim.

Yes, the bags are another investment consideration. However, you'll end up producing more of a better-quality base product than with the coffee pad option, which is the 2nd option. Let me walk you through the Bubble bag procedure first. The two methods are similar, with the 2nd one being only a slight variation on the 1st.

With the Bubble bag method, you'll be using multiple filtration bags of varying sized screens to sort the resinous glands into grades. As previously mentioned, a 4-bag set of extraction Bubble Bags will cost about $25 US.

The process is a simple one to understand. By freezing your plant material, the resin-coated trichomes become brittle and they can be easily separated from the organic matter. Ice water is used to transport the wet kief through each successive layer of bags. The wet kief trapped on the screen of each bag can then be scraped off using a spoon and placed on a sheet of clean cardboard for drying.

Here's an 8-step process to producing water hash:
Step #1: Get your buds and trim ready. At least one day before you decide to make your water hash, pick up (or make) a bag of ice. And place your bud and trim you'll be processing in plastic freezer bags and pop them into the freezer. I also like to place a 1-gallon water jug of reverse osmosis water in the refrigerator to cool it down.

Step #2: Set up your equipment. On water hash day, start by washing your Bubble bags thoroughly with clean water. Beg, borrow or steal an electric drill along with a dough hook that's typically used with a hand mixer. The drill and dough hook combination make it easy to mix your ice slurry.

Also have a pair of surgical gloves, water spray bottle, tablespoon, knife, and set of mixing bowls handy. The spray bottle and spoon come in handy when collecting your water-logged kief for drying. Try to find a mixing bowl or another type of container that you can stretch your Bubble bags over. I use a small, circular, one-foot high garbage can at home. Don't worry, it's clean.

Step #3: Set up your Bubble bags. Stretch your clean Bubble bags over your container. The outermost bag (first layer) will be the one with the smallest micron screen (73 micron). Layer your bags one inside the other ending up with the largest diameter screen on top (220 micron). This first layer traps large organic matter. The subsequent layers capture finer and finer grades of water hash.

Step #4: Mix your ice/cannabis slurry together. Fill your Bubble bag container 3/4 full, with alternating layers of ice, cold water and frozen material. Using the dough hook drill set-up, agitate your slurry for 15 minutes. You may wish to wear ear plugs or hearing protection while the drill is whirling. This process knocks off the frozen trichomes on your material, which will pass through successive layers of your bags.

Go for coffee. Seriously, take a 15-minute break before moving on to step #5. After agitating the crap-ola out of your material, let it sit and settle undisturbed.

Step #5: Remove the water and organic material. Carefully lift your bags from the ice water. Allow time for most of the water to slowly drain from the bags. Then, gently squeeze any remaining water out of your Bubble bag combo while wearing your gloves. Once most of the water has been removed, separate the first bag containing most of the organic material and set this aside for a possible 2nd extraction. You'll end of with a series of bags containing finer and finer grades of water hash after that initial organic matter bag.

Step #6: Spray down and remove the water hash. Stretch the first bag containing water hash over a mixing bowl or other container so that it exposes the water hash on the screening material. Using your spray bottle and a spoon, gently spray and scrape the hash towards the center of the screen. Remove the clump of water hash with your spoon and place it onto the cardboard sheet. As well, I like to use a small curved knife to scrape down my spoon. Try to spread the water hash out to form a thin, even, pancake layer. You may notice that this hash has a slight green tinge to it as it contains a small amount of vegetative matter.

Repeat this process with each successive layer of bags. You'll discover that each layer of water hash will change in color from light green to a golden yellow. This indicates that the finer bag layers are screening out a higher grade of wet kief.

Step #7: Repeat the process. Repeat steps #3 to #6 using the remaining material you would like to process. As a final step, you could process some of the remaining organic material a second time to extract any remaining trichomes that weren't removed the first go around.

Step #8: Dry your water hash. Using the cardboard as a drying platform, place it in a dry, room temperature environment overnight. I usually just pop mine back into the grow tent after it has been cleaned. Then, I'll run both the inline and desk fans to remove odors and built up humidity. Also, cover the hash with a clean paper towel so dust doesn't contaminate it. At least once over the next 24-hour period, flip your hash cake over so that it dries out evenly from both sides.

The coffee filter method:

This method is slightly less expensive than using Bubble bags, assuming that you have some of the kitchen gadgets needed for the processing.

Many of the Bubble bag method steps are identical to the coffee filter method. Here's an 8-step process to producing water hash using coffee filters and kitchen tools:

Step #1: Get your buds and trim ready. A day or so before you make your water hash make or buy a bag of ice. Place your bud and trim you'll be processing in plastic freezer bags and pop them into the freezer overnight. Also, have a 1-gallon water jug of cold reverse osmosis water ready as well.

Step #2: Set up your equipment. On water hash day, set aside a blender, mixing bowl, fine wire mesh strainer, reusable cone-shaped coffee filter, several cone-type paper coffee filters, 2 or 3 large glass jars with tight-sealing lids (mason jars), a spoon, a small curved knife and a pair of surgical gloves.

Step #3: Grind your material. Layer your ice, cold water and plant material in equal parts in the blender. Turn on the blender at full speed for 1 minute. You may want to wear hearing protection. Let the material settle for 1 minute. Repeat the process 3 times.

Step #4: Strain the organic material. Using the wire mesh strainer and mixing bowl, strain your slurry. Pour the green-tinted water through the reusable cone-shaped coffee filter into quart-size jars until full. The resinous trichomes have passed through both the wire screen and initial coffee filter into the jars.

Step #5: Cool down and settle out the water hash. Place each of the jars in the refrigerator for 1 hour. The resinous trichomes will settle out and form a silt at the bottom of each jar.

Step #6: Separate the water hash from the water. Without disturbing your sediment, carefully remove the jars from the fridge. Slowly pour off the top portion of the water, while retaining the water hash. You'll end up with a slurry of hash along with a small amount of water.

Step #7: Strain your water hash. Set up a disposable paper coffee filter on a jar. Slowly pour the slurry into the filter. Better yet, use a section of clean flexible aquarium tubing to siphon off the top water layer. The siphon provides greater control and generates less turbulence in the water. Retain the water hash collected on the paper filter.

Step #8: Dry your water hash. Flatten out your coffee filter on a cloth or paper towel to absorb most of the water. Then place it on a flat tray or container in a dry, room-temperature, environment overnight. Continue drying and curing your hash as outlined in the first water hash method. If you have a seedling propagation heating mat (some hot houses come with one), use it to dry the water hash. You could even use a food dehydrator that is set on low to dry the hash faster.

Taking the time to prepare water hash has some distinct benefits, namely:
1. It helps to rinse any chemical residues off the plant material, resulting in a cleaner final product.
2. The water hash can be easily incorporated into a variety of products, such as edibles, tinctures and ointments.
3. The dried hash takes up very little storage space making it easier to be discreet about your consumption.

Water hash often tests out as containing 50% cannabinoids, which is an impressive level of quality. As a rule of thumb, expect to produce 3g of hash for every 30 g of bud and shake.

Once the hash cake is dry to the touch, you can either prep it for storage or for further processing. I usually discombobulate … I mean decarboxylate the hash at this point in time.

What the heck is decarboxylation and why is it so important?

Growing cannabis plants contain the acidic form of CBD and THC, known as CBDA and THCA. A carbonate molecule (COOH) is attached to the cannabinoids making them only marginally active. Decarboxylation is the process of using heat to remove the carbonate molecule and create the active forms of CBD and THC.

When you smoke/ vape marijuana, CBDA and THCA are converted to active forms as the marijuana is burned or heated during vaping. The same holds true for marijuana that is used in the cooking process.

Your water hash is in the inactive form. It needs to be heated in order to be used in certain edible products, tinctures and ointments.

Here's a three-step process for decarboxylating your water hash:

1. You'll need to set up the following items: parchment paper, aluminum foil, cookie baking tray, knife, oven thermometer, oven/ toaster oven. Now set your oven to 240°F with the oven thermometer visible inside. This is the ideal temperature for CBDA-rich hash. As a side note, THCA should be decarboxylated at a slightly cooler temperature of 220°F.

2. Thoroughly break up your hash into fine pieces or powder. Place the hash on 1/2 of a sheet of aluminum foil. Loosely fold the other half over to protect it from dispersing in the air. Carefully place the aluminum foil sandwich onto the cookie sheet.

3. Place your cookie sheet into the pre-heated oven or toaster and set a timer for 40 minutes. You may need to adjust the temperature during the baking process so that it hovers within a 5°F range. At a minimum, bake your hash for at least 30 minutes to achieve optimal levels of CBD and THC conversion.

After removing your decarboxylated hash from the oven, allow it to cool completely before storing. This process can produce some strong odors. Setting up your inline fan and carbon filter and/or using odor absorbing gels like Ona Gel can help eliminate most of these odors.

Now that we have the raw material for producing a myriad of beneficial products, let's look at several ways of converting your water hash into an assortment of common forms. The forms you'll be shown are:

1. Infused Vegetable Oils and Butter.
2. Alcohol and Glycerin Tinctures.
3. Canna-cap Capsules.
4. Topical Salves.
5. CBD Oil (Rick Simpson Oil).

For most of the following procedures, you'll be using decarboxylated hash. If the heating process is short and at a low temperature, this is the case.

I've listed these five classes of products in order of preparation difficulty from easiest to more challenging projects. Let's begin by creating some oils and butters for the kitchen.

How to make infused vegetable oils and butter.

Cannabis-infused cooking oils are easy to make, store and use. Coconut, olive, flaxseed and canola are all good choices.

Let's take a look at the cooking oil process:

Step #1: Set up your equipment. You'll need a double boiler, a spatula, an emersion thermometer, a paper coffee filter, a glass storage bottle, 8 to 16 ounces of oil, and a small quantity of finely-ground, decarboxylated hash (0.5 to 1 gram).

Step #2: Combine your ingredients. Start by heating the water in your double boiler to 100°F - 125°F. Keeping the temperature low decreases the chances of heat degradation occurring. Add the cooking oil. Once warmed, add the ground hash, stirring to dissolve.

Step #3: Stir hourly. Over the course of the next 4 to 6 hours stir your mixture. Add warm water to your double boiler hourly.

Step #4: Cool and store. Allow the oil to cool. Then pour it through the coffee filter into a labeled, empty, glass bottle suitable for oils. Refrigerate immediately.

These oils can be used at low temperatures in your favorite recipes. Unfortunately, high temperature frying or cooking, will destroy most of the cannabinoids.

Virtually the same process can be used to create canna-butter. Start with 1/2 pound of butter and the same quantity of finely ground hash. Follow the same process above with the exception of simmering the butter mixture for only 45 minutes and avoiding the use of a coffee filter in the final step.

Should you find the taste a bit offensive, try adding fresh herbs like basil or cilantro, or a touch of lime or lemon juice and zest to the mixture. You could even mince a clove of garlic along with some finely chopped parsley to make garlic butter. Get creative!

How to make alcohol and glycerine tinctures.

How do you make alcohol-based tinctures that'll make mama proud? Alcohol-based tinctures are easy to create with your decarboxylated hash and they can be stored for months, even years with proper care since alcohol is a great preservative.

The tinctures can be administered under the tongue sublingually with an eyedropper for faster absorption into the bloodstream. Dosing becomes easier and more consistent when using tinctures. The tincture can be added to coffee, juice or another beverage to make it more palatable.

Here's a step-by-step alcohol-based process to follow:

Step #1: Purchase a bottle high proof alcohol. Buy a bottle of 190-proof alcohol like Everclear (where available), 151-proof Bacardi rum or 192-proof Spirytus Polish vodka. The higher the alcohol concentration, the easier it is to dissolve your hash. At a minimum use 80-proof (40%) alcohol.

Step #2: Prep your materials. Pour your alcohol into a clean glass jar with a resealable lid. We like to use 1-quart mason jars. Grind 0.5 to 2 grams of decarboxylated hash as fine as possible, thus making it easier to dissolve in the alcohol. You could use a mortar and pestle or break the hash up using a fine-bladed knife. Then, add it to the alcohol.

Step #3: Shake your jar daily. Over the course of the next week to 10 days, shake the contents of your jar on a daily basis to help dissolve the hash. Keep your jar in a warm, dark spot. Ten days is usually sufficient time when working with hash. A longer soak time extracts more cannabinoids and essential oils. Should you be using buds or trim, allow the mixture to sit at least 3 to 4 weeks.

Step #4: Filter your solution. Using a paper coffee filter, strain any solid material through the filter. Retain the residue, which can be dried and used for vaping or cooking later. What you'll end up with in the jar is a CBD-rich alcohol-based tincture.

For those who don't like the taste or want to use alcohol, glycerin tinctures are an alternative. The best method is to prepare an alcohol tincture first, then add it to the glycerin. Since cannabis is less soluble in glycerin than alcohol, starting with an alcohol-based tincture produces a more potent end product. You can pick up an inexpensive bottle of pure USP-grade glycerin at your local drugstore or online.

Here's the alcohol/ glycerin process in detail:

Step #1: Set up your equipment. You'll need a double boiler, rice cooker or crock pot set on its lowest temperature. Set up your equipment in a well-ventilated area away from any open flames. You'll also need your alcohol-based tincture, a spatula and glass storage jar with resealable top.

Step #2: Combine the ingredients. Pour your tincture into your pot along with an almost equal amount of glycerin. Limit the depth of your mixture to just a few inches. Start up your pot. Using your spatula blend the two ingredients while maintaining a low temperature setting. The alcohol will evaporate. Once you can no longer smell the alcohol, your tincture is done.

Step #3: Transfer your tincture. Carefully transfer your glycerin-based tincture into a clean jar. Don't strain your tincture through a paper filter. It will clog. Allow it to cool to room temperature before sealing, then place it in the fridge for long-term storage. Glycerin tinctures spoil in a few weeks if not refrigerated.

How to make canna-cap capsules.

Canna caps are edible gelatin-filled capsules that contain a small dose of cannabis. Vegetarian capsules made of starch can also be purchased. These capsules can be filled with:
1. dry powder containing kief,
2. hash mixed with an oil, or
3. oil extract made from hash.

The most popular form is to mix hash with coconut oil. Why coconut oil you may ask? Coconut oil is a solid at normal room temperature, which makes it easier to prepare and use. Since we'll be storing the canna caps in the fridge, the coconut oil solidifies, making it easier to handle when you're feeling the urge.

What you'll require are the following items:
1. capsule filling machine, which is available at many health food stores or online. Look for a size #0 machine. This is the smallest size available. Being small in size, your capsules are easier to swallow, and the dosage is easier to regulate.
2. 50 to 60 gelatin or vegetarian size #0 capsules,
3. electronic scale accurate to 0.5 grams,
4. double boiler,
5. mixing spoon,
6. coconut oil (28 grams or 1 ounce),
7. large syringe (10 cc),
8. small quantity of finely-ground decarboxylated hash (2.0 grams or 0.07 ounces),
9. relatively airtight storage container like an old vitamin bottle.

Each capsule can hold up to 0.3 grams of product. Using 2.0 grams of hash and 28 grams of oil will give you about 100 capsules. I've found that this recipe allows you to more easily adjust your dosage. If one capsule isn't enough, two may be what the doctor orders.

The capsule machines have a platform with holes into which you place the bottom half of your capsules. By using a large syringe, you can inject the oil/ hash mixture into each capsule. Then seal each capsule with the top half.

Here's a blow by blow description of how to make a mess in your kitchen:
Step #1: Set up your equipment. Have everything listed above ready to go. Also, set up your canna cap machine with your capsules. Start by heating the water in your double boiler to 100°F - 125°F so that the oil and hash can dissolve slowly in a warm bath.

*Step #2: **Weigh out your oil and hash**.* Add your oil to the double boiler. Add your ground hash after the oil has heated up. Continually stir your mixture for several minutes to help dissolve the hash in the oil.

*Step #3: **Heat your mixture**.* Periodically stir your mixture over the span of 30 to 60 minutes in an attempt to have as much hash dissolved in the oil as possible. A long slow heating process results in a more homogeneous mixture.

*Step #4: **Allow your mixture to cool slightly**.* Remove your cannabis oil mixture from the heat and allow it to cool slightly so that you can draw it up into your syringe or pour it into your capsules without being rushed to the hospital with 2nd degree burns.

*Step #5: **Fill each capsule**.* Using a syringe or very, very, careful pouring, fill the bottom of each canna cap that you've previously loaded into the filling machine. Place the top cap onto each filled capsule, pressing gently until you feel it lock into place.

*Step #6: **Rinse and repeat**.* Once the canna caps are relatively cool to the touch, place them in your storage container and pop them into the fridge. Repeat this whole process with a second batch of capsules.

And there you have it. Medicine to be used as needed.

How to make cannabis salves.

Topical salves that are applied to the skin help with joint pain and localized inflammation. To make a topical salve, we'll be blending a small amount of your hash with oil and beeswax. Some fast-absorbing oils to consider using are coconut and grape-seed. You could also use glycerin instead of oil. To kick up your salve a notch, consider adding ingredients like menthol, echinacea, ichthammol, calendula and vitamin E in small amounts. Not only do many of these adjuncts smell good, they also offer some therapeutic benefits.

Here's how to create your topical salve:
*Step #1: **Set aside your equipment**.*
You'll need:

1. double boiler,
2. electronic scale to measure out your ingredients,
3. 1 gram (0.04 ounces) of finely-ground, decarboxylated hash,
4. 500 ml (~1 pint) of oil,
5. 42 grams (1.5 ounces) of beeswax,
6. mixing spoon,
7. wide-mouthed glass storage jars and
8. any essential oils you would like to add at the very end of the process.

Fire up your double boiler or stainless-steel crock pot and try to keep the temperature below 125°F. Recall, that we want to use low heat to help dissolve the ingredients without drastically altering the cannabinoids with excessive heat.

Step #2: Dissolve the hash in your oil. Add the oil to the pot and allow the mixture to come together over the course of the next 30 to 60 minutes with occasional stirring at a low temperature.

Step #3: Add the beeswax. If you're using finely ground hash, you shouldn't have to strain out any solid material that is typically left over if you were using dried buds. Add the majority of the beeswax to your mixture, allowing it to dissolve.

Step #4: Test for doneness. Using your spoon, set aside a spoonful to cool for several minutes. Using your fingers, test your salve for hardness. If it is too soft add more beeswax to the mix. Repeat the process until your desired consistency is reached.

Step #5: Add any essential oils or vitamin E. Once you have a firm enough salve, add a small portion of any additional ingredients to the mix.

Step #6: Prep for storage. Pour your liquid salve into wide-mouthed glass storage jars. Label and place your jars in the fridge for long-term storage.

Besides cannabis salves, you can also prepare topical lotions that use the above recipe with an added step. Once you complete step #5, slowly add small quantities of distilled or reverse osmosis water to the mix while using a hand-held mixer set on low speed. You want to emulsify the entire mixture to make it fluffy. You can then transfer your lotion into a bottle for future use once it has cooled slightly.

How to make CBD oil (Rick Simpson oil).

Recall that Rich Simpson gained notoriety back in the late 90's when he began growing cannabis and producing cannabis oil for the treatment of cancer and other ailments. Rick Simpson Oil is named after this Canadian medical marijuana activist.

The process described below is a twist on Rick's classic recipe. Instead of using isopropyl alcohol or another toxic solvent, we'll be using drinking or ethyl alcohol. And instead of starting with dried bud (which is always an option), we'll be using our dried water hash. No need to use decarboxylated hash as this process will do it for you.

Following the method outlined below, produces a better-quality CBD-rich oil than trying to buy a bushel of hemp and processing it yourself to extract a minute amount of CBD. Granted, commercial production of "hemp oil" may be a viable option on a grand scale. However, for the home grower it isn't pragmatic, since hemp contains very low concentration levels of cannabinoids. CBD-rich hash or dried bud are much better alternatives.

Without further ado, here's how to make Rick Simpson CBD oil without blowing up the house:

Step #1: Set up your equipment. Since you'll be evaporating alcohol during the cooking process, a well-ventilated room with no open flames is a must. You may wish to set up your inline fan and carbon filter to help control both the odor and air flow. Setting up a desk fan that blows the fumes away from the heating source is also advisable. You'll need:

1. rice cooker,
2. desk fan and/or inline fan with carbon filter,
3. 500 mL (~ 1 pint) of high-proof drinking alcohol (Everclear or Spirytus Polish Vodka),

183

4. 3 grams (0.1 ounces) of finely ground water hash,
5. electronic scale to measure out the hash,
6. spatula or spoon for stirring,
7. several 10 cc plastic syringes for the final oil,
8. 1/2 teaspoon of water,
9. oven mitts.

Step #2: *Combine the alcohol and hash*. Add the alcohol and hash to your rice cooker without the lid on. Stir the mixture for several minutes to begin the assimilation process. Turn on your rice cooker. Constantly stir the mixture as the rice cooker heats up to help dissolve the hash. Continue heating and occasionally stirring for 1 to 3 hours.

Step #3: *Add the water*. At sea level, water boils at 212°F, whereas alcohol boils at 173°F. Adding water at the end of alcohol evaporation, allows the alcohol to be released as it thickens without burning your oil. Once you get to this point of the process, pick up your rice cooker with your oven mitts and swirl the final contents to release the alcohol and prevent the oil from burning.

Step #4: *Remove the water*. When you have a thick dark oil, remove the pot from the rice cooker. Carefully pour the mixture into a metal measuring cup and place this on a gentle heating surface like a coffee warmer or place the cup in a dehydrator. Allow the water left in the mixture to evaporate over the course of a couple of hours. Once any bubbling ceases, it's ready for storage.

Step #5: *Fill your syringes*. Set the oil aside to cool slightly. Once cool enough, use the syringes to draw the vicious oil up into each syringe. Store them in the fridge once done.

You now have a better idea as to how you could grow and produce an assortment of CBD-rich products that'll improve the quality of your life.

From learning how to become a do-it-yourself grower, let's explore how you could become a do-it-yourself investor in the ever-evolving cannabis industry. Time for a well-deserved break before we take a look at how to invest in cannabis in the next section. Wouldn't you agree?

Section 4: How to Profit from the Cannabis Industry.

Very little has been written about how you could benefit financially from the cannabis industry in North America. In this last section you'll learn about:

1.What current and future job opportunities are out there that you could capitalize on.

2. What business and investment opportunities could put more money into your piggy bank.

4. Why you should become a do-it-yourself stock investor and how to do it so that you take advantage of our tax system.

4. Why you should become a "cash flow" stock investor.

5. How to build an additional monthly income stream by "renting" out cannabis stock (or any other stock) that you own.

6. How to initially find wonderful stocks to invest in.

7. How to quickly assess the potential profitability of a company.

8. How to select the "right" investment strategy that'll generate a monthly stream of income.

9. How to time when to enter and exit positions.

Let's begin by exploring a variety of employment and business opportunities in this fast-growing industry.

Chapter 8: What Employment & Investment Opportunities Are There?

Why invest in the cannabis industry?

There is a growing international movement of making cannabis available to more and more medical patients who could take advantage of the therapeutic benefits of cannabinoids. We're also seeing more and more countries legalizing the use of recreational marijuana and de-criminalizing the possession of marijuana. For example, Canada has recently legalized the recreational use of marijuana and Mexico is slated to follow suit. This opens up the door for big business and local governments to profit from the production, distribution and sale of a variety of cannabis-related products.

In 2017, legal marijuana sales in the US alone topped out at over $10 billion. The Canadian market is expected to surpass $5 billion by 2020 in domestic and international sales. There are over 30,000 legal marijuana-based businesses across North America. And the United States Marijuana Index, a cannabis stock index, is currently valued at over $5.5 billion. There's no denying that cannabis is a lucrative business. Wouldn't you want a piece of this action?

Despite the US government's tight control over research, trade and access, many jurisdictions have taken the underground cannabis movement and legitimized the market. Local governments everywhere want a piece of this lucrative pie. So, why not invest in the business of the production and distribution of cannabis and cannabis-related products?

Many local governments are tapping into the taxation revenue streams that the industry offers, not unlike the alcohol and tobacco sectors. More than 1/2 of the States in the US have laws in place for the medical and/or recreational use of marijuana. And big business sees the cannabis industry as a multi-billion, dollar cash cow waiting to be milked for decades to come.

As entire countries begin to legalize the industry, these countries are now capable of gearing up production on a global scale of cannabis-related products. Making it lucrative for both the government and major international corporations.

Employment opportunities:

As the cannabis industry evolves innovative ways of bringing an assortment of cannabis-related products to the general public has also mushroomed. Jobs in sectors that didn't exist just a few years ago are popping up all over the country. If you're considering employment within the cannabis industry, there is no better time than now to find meaningful employment. Here's a smattering of some area where rapid growth is occurring.

Employment within the Industry:

There is a growing demand for individuals who have certain skill sets and post-secondary education training in disciplines related to bio-chemistry, agriculture, engineering, and food science.

As more production facilities are being built, whether they be greenhouses, self-contained indoor growing facilities or outdoor venues, skilled laborers are needed for the initial construction, continued maintenance and on-going production.

Cannabis grown indoors is labor intensive, requiring constant monitoring and attentive care in order to produce consistent, high-yield crops every 4 to 6 months. This opens up the door for individuals to work year-round in many facilities that seem to be popping up everywhere.

For example, Cannabis Wheaton in partnership with GreenhouseCo, plans to build a 1.4 million square foot greenhouse that'll produce 120,000 kilograms of cannabis per year. And Canopy Growth in partnership with Tweed has converted an old Hershey Chocolate factory into a 168,000 square foot indoor facility capable of producing 6,000 kilograms of cannabis. Both of these massive facilities need skilled and trained workers.

Besides the cultivation aspect of the business, post-production job opportunities abound. Manufacturers are looking for individuals who can convert the raw material into edible products, infused beverages, lotions, capsules, tinctures and a host of other health-related products.

Many spin-off sectors are also growing. The move towards providing pesticide and chemical free, clean bud requires testing services of labs equipped to analyze marijuana. As more government-regulated, growing facilities come on board, the need for testing also increases. This means more job opportunities in this sector alone.

One of the largest beverage companies in the world, Constellation Brands, has entered into an agreement with Canopy Growth to eventually produce a wide assortment of cannabis infused non-alcoholic and alcoholic beverages.

Big business is gearing up for the world-wide distribution of cannabis-related products. Isn't it about time you considered the possibilities?

Take compassion clubs and local retailers for example. Compassion clubs typically serve medical marijuana users. These organizations often hire individuals from the health-care sector who understand the benefits and use of cannabis-related products. And local retailers are always looking for knowledgeable sales staff who can promote certain products and services.

Employment within Local Government:

Positions are being created in many jurisdictions that did not exist just a few years ago. As these jurisdictions tap into the revenue stream that the cannabis industry can provide through taxation or government-controlled production and distribution facilities, new positions need to be created to manage these new portfolios.

As more and more states and provinces gear up for legalization, local governments will require more staff dedicated to managing, regulating, and enforcing policies.

Both managerial and front-line positions will be needed to administer the day-to-day tasks that'll keep the entire system running smoothly.

Employment within Post-Secondary Institutions:

More and more colleges are now offering entire programs geared towards the cannabis industry. Should you already have a desirable skill set, this may be your ticket.

If not, you could look at this sector as an educational opportunity to become more marketable with a skill set geared to the growing number of jobs being offered. If the cannabis industry develops anything like the wine industry, you'll see programs geared specifically to cultivation, production and marketing.

Business opportunities:

Are you an entrepreneur? Then, look to spin-off industries for business opportunities. Sure, you could try to compete with the big boys by becoming a grower. However, more and more small grow ops are being gobbled up by big business.

Not to mention that marijuana production is becoming less profitable unless you've got economies of scale working for you. Massive growing facilities are able to lower production costs substantially. For example, in Washington State where recreational and medical marijuana are legal, the price of 1 gram of cannabis has dropped over a 3-year period since 2015 from an average retail price of $10 to close to $7. This reduction also takes into consideration the 37% excise tax being imposed on cannabis sales. This means that the little guy is having a harder time to compete as the commodity drops in price. Breeders and growers are becoming more efficient in producing high-grade, cost-effective marijuana products.

Your best bet is to look at business opportunities that target specific sectors that support the cultivation sector. This could be businesses that use cannabis to produce edible products, beverages, health care creams and lotions, capsules and pills, or tinctures, to name a few.

It could also be sectors that support the overall industry, such as graphic design, product packaging, quality control, marketing, or even seed production labs. Each of these business opportunities taps into a skill set that is in growing demand.

And what about the growing need of retail businesses that sell grow op equipment and supplies. No pun intended. Well, maybe, just a little bit. We're seeing increased equipment sales for setting up small-scale grow ops in homes, especially in jurisdictions where the personal cultivation of marijuana plants has become legal.

There's also a need for nutritional products and systems geared specifically for growing marijuana. And what about consultation services for the general public. With growing demand there are all sorts of business opportunities.

Could you see yourself working in the industry down the road? Let's look at how you could tap into this lucrative industry right now by looking at how you could invest in the industry leaders.

Chapter 9: Why Should I Become a Cash Flow Investor?

If you want immediate access to the profit stream that major corporations are benefitting from now and into the future, then the stock market is your answer.

Before we delve into seven mega-trends that could be profitable to you down the road, let's explore how you could optimize your stock market gains, while protecting your capital. What you're about to learn is going to change your whole perspective about stock investing. No longer will you fear the wide swings of the market that are a part of our normal economic cycle.

Fundamental to every investment portfolio is protecting your hard-earned capital. You're going to learn how to both protect your stock investments, as well as generate a monthly stream of cash by renting out your stock.

Yes ... renting out your stock. It's no different than owning a rental property and collecting monthly rent from your renters.

I'll show you how you can safely invest in the markets with some simple, tried and true strategies. But before we get to that, let's take a look at what a "typical" stock market investor can expect.

Stock market reality check.

The vast majority of stock market investors place their hard-earned dollars in the hands of a trusted mutual fund advisor, which is the traditional approach to investing in the markets. Many well-intentioned investors who followed the advice of their mutual fund advisers lost a substantial portion of their hard-earned capital during the stock market crashes of 2001 and 2008. You may have seen your portfolio decimated in the wake of these two, major, set-backs.

Many of these passive investors panicked, moving their money out of stocks and into cash or bonds, right when the markets started to rebound missing yet another opportunity to grow their investment portfolios. It does not take much to see that this collective ignorance has a long-term negative impact on one's ability to build wealth.

You may be asking yourself why bother trying to invest when I can't even get ahead. It will take me another 20 to 30 years to get back to even if a use a buy and hold - and pray approach to investing in the markets. I don't have this much time if I'm approaching retirement. And just as I think I've made some progress, I get hit by another market meltdown and my portfolio suffers yet another blow. How can I even fathom regaining control over my investments? Sound familiar to you or someone you know?

I recall, a close colleague of mine during my public-school teaching days foaming at the mouth as he expressed his frustration with his mutual fund advisor. His advisor had him switching from one fund to another over a 10-year period, chasing after returns. It was driving him up the wall. His overall portfolio grew only by the additional deposits he had made over the years. He was bitter about what was unfolding and felt at a loss over what he could do.

I too would be frustrated and disillusioned with a system that was supposed to build my wealth over time. What's even more aggravating are the lies that the financial services industry has been perpetrating over the decades about investing in the stock market.

Many mutual fund advisers and financial advisers tout that stocks in the S&P 500 Index have generated an average return of around 10% over the past 90 years. This lulls investors into thinking that the stock market produces consistently high returns with little or no volatility. However, they don't tell you that markets do not climb upwards in a straight line. The very nature of the stock market is that it is subject to wild swings, not unlike the waves of the ocean during a storm.

The fact is - average returns are not average and much less so today. Markets have changed due to a surge in equity and commodity volatility and uncertainty. Relying on old rules is a recipe for disaster.

According to **James O'Shaughnessy** in his classic guide to the best-performing investment strategies of all time **What Works on Wall Street**: *"Seventy percent of the mutual funds covered by Morningstar fail to beat the S&P 500 over almost any 10-year period because their managers lack the discipline to stick with one strategy. This lack of discipline devastates long-term performance."*

So, why is it that some actively-engaged investors are able to generate double digit returns on their money in the stock market in a year like 2011, yet most mutual fund investors lost money over the same period?

In 2011 the S&P 500 Index started and ended the year flat with no appreciable gains and most mutual fund investors ended up with a loss at year's end. However, a little stock investment knowledge allows the informed active investor great wealth creation opportunities despite what the markets were doing.

Watching your investment portfolio being decimated by the markets and not knowing how you can capitalize on great investment opportunities as they unfold is both disheartening and discouraging. You may feel completely at a loss and totally helpless in not being able to do a thing about your investments when the normal market volatility takes its toll on your holdings. Panic may set in. And in the heat of panic you may move out of positions only to realize that you've once again missed a great opportunity.

This deception about how the markets really function is often not taken into consideration in one's overall investment plan, especially in the short term. Without truly knowing how the markets function you are unable to incorporate money-making strategies that capitalize on the normal fluctuations of the stock market. This is what you'll learn how to do by the end of this book - on my boy scout's honor.

What do all wealth builders do?

The majority of self-made millionaires focus their time and energy on three types of smart investments, namely:

1. Their ongoing financial education in specific areas that will have a direct impact on their ability to grow their capital under all market conditions.
2. Their ability to acquire cash flowing assets, whether it be in the stock market, real estate or certain commodities.
3. Their ability to build systematized businesses that are able to generate passive income while they sleep.

Let's take a quick look at each of these smart investment vehicles and how they might help you down the road.

Vehicle #1: Become Financially Intelligent.

By picking up a copy of this book, you have taken the first step to building your knowledge so that you can profit from all that the cannabis industry has to offer. Your curiosity has paid off. It has been a motivational factor in moving you closer to realizing your desires and maybe even your dreams.

Did you know that it's more and more challenging to pursue the American Dream? Why? Because you have to be asleep to believe it.

You on the other hand have stepped from the realm of the "wanna be" wealth dreamer who is all talk and no action - to having made a conscious decision to actually do something about your financial affairs. You're reading this section right now, aren't you?

Now it's time to start creating wealth for you and your loved ones. And, it all begins with the most important tool that you can develop - your financial intelligence.

Increasing your financial intelligence over time will empower you to solve the money problems that you may be faced with at this moment. By improving the quality of the financial information that you use in your decision-making and differentiating between fact and opinion you set yourself up to be in a better position to tap into your financial genius.

Vehicle #2: Acquire Assets.

The second smart investment vehicle is to acquire assets that put money into your pockets. In other words, invest in those asset classes with a proven track record of generating cash flow from the investment.

The top three general asset classes that most people are familiar with as investment opportunities are equities, real estate and commodities. This section of the book delves into the world of stock investing and shows you step-by-step how to implement an accelerated cash flow investment system that systematically puts money into your pocket.

The second general asset class that active investors like to invest in is real estate. A common cash flow approach in real estate is to buy an investment property and then rent it out as a means of generating a monthly income. Coincidentally, this is similar to the covered call strategy of "renting out" your stock in the options market, whereby you receive a monthly cash premium for doing so.

And finally, the third asset class is that of investing in commodities such as oil wells, precious metal mines or alternative energy ventures that can provide a monthly check.

Each of these asset classes has specific benefits, risks and rewards.

For most investors who are trying to build their wealth, the most cost-effective and time-efficient way to generate cash flow is through the stock market. As your wealth begins to accumulate, you may wish to further explore investing in rental real estate or specific commodity plays since these investment classes tend to be a little more capital intensive to start off with.

Whether you choose equities, real estate or commodities as your preferred asset class, please keep in mind that your focus should be on putting money into your pocket through positive cash flow. If most of the stock analysts look favorably upon those businesses that have the ability to generate ongoing cash flow, why wouldn't you want to emulate what they value most - an increasing stream of incoming cash?

195

Vehicle #3: Build Systematized Businesses.

I mention the third smart investment vehicle, only to give you a complete perspective of the three major areas where the resources of effective wealth builders can be allocated for creating sustainable wealth.

For the highly motivated individual, the option of building a low-start-up cost, systematized business that runs on its own even when you're not present is appealing. It's definitely one effective way to exit the rat race from a 9 to 5 job, be the master of your own destiny and not succumb to your employer's chosen path for you. And the growing cannabis industry provides many an entrepreneur with business opportunities.

A word of caution though - be aware that starting any business requires hard work and patience. Don't confuse "get rich quick", which is a distinct possibly for you, with "get rich easy". Unfortunately, there are too many self-promoting experts who'll tell you differently, especially those that are flaunting a particular product or service. Over the years I have come across several online marketers who have been touting the same message:" Blogging is easy. I'll show you how to get a blog up and running in less than one hour and then you'll see the money rolling in." Don't let anyone try to fool you into thinking that building any business is easy.

Of course, on the flip side of this coin is the wealth creation potential that you can tap into should you have realistic expectations and develop an appropriate business attitude that factors in the amount of time and effort required to build your second or third stream of income. Makes sense, right?

Insights to Consider:

Having an understanding of these three smart investing options in the back of your mind, you'll begin to assess opportunities and make money allocation decisions in a different light.

For example, my wife and I have come to an understanding that our hard-earned dollars are channeled into investments that either improve our level of financial education or purchase an appreciating cash flowing asset. When we have appropriately allocated our monetary resources towards building our dreams, it provides us with a greater sense of accomplishment, confidence, ongoing motivation and hope for a better future for the two of us.

You too can walk a similar path to financial freedom.

Now that you have an idea as to where you can channel your future efforts, let's take a look at what you need in order to succeed as a cash flow investor.

Tap into these three wealth pillars:

I also came to understand that in order to build sustainable wealth over time; I needed to channel my efforts into three specific areas, which I call my wealth pillars.

Pillar #1: Increasing my savings for investment purposes.

Everything hinges on the first pillar. If you do not make saving for investing a priority - you cannot invest - if you cannot invest - you cannot create the lifestyle that you dream about. During the course of this section of the book, we'll explore several simple approaches that'll get you headed in the right direction. The first pillar to wealth creation remains your ability to move capital into investment opportunities as a result of your saving to invest regime.

Pillar #2: Investing in "Best of Breed" stocks.

As you will see, this pillar will become a structural part of your wealth creation machine. Buying stock of those businesses that are the market leaders in their sector lends itself to a higher probability that the shares will appreciate in value more so than average stocks in that sector. The market likes businesses that have solid growth in earnings and cash flow. And we like cannabis stocks that show promising international growth.

Pillar #3: Selling option contracts on stock that you own.

This pillar piggy backs off of the previous one. In essence, you receive a cash premium in your brokerage account when you agree to sell your stock shares at a specific price on or before a pre-determined date.

I'll show you how you can generate a monthly flow of cash into your account, by renting out your stock similar to how a property owner rents out an apartment unit. The process of selling covered calls can generate a conservative monthly cash flow of 2 to 3 percent when properly structured, which is what you'll learn more about by the end of this section.

Why you too can do it!

The average knowledgeable investor can follow in my footsteps, or those of the experts who are showcased in this resource and do exactly what I have been so fortunate to realize. By learning how to use simple investment strategies coupled with time-tested approaches, you'll be able to head down the path to financial freedom that'll eventually lead to fulfilling your dreams.

You may be asking yourself: So, if these strategies can consistently produce double digit returns over the long haul why don't more people follow a similar system? Why aren't more people getting rich from investing in the stock market?

Which brings us to the most destructive myths in the financial service industry that dissuade people from acting and becoming cash flow generating machines in the stock market.

The two biggest financial myths holding you back:

Myth #1: You need over $1 million to retire comfortably.
Unfortunately, we've all been brain-washed into thinking that we need to amass a huge nest egg in order to live comfortably during our retirement years. This assumes that we move our investment capital into more conservative investment vehicles such as bonds, treasury notes or certificates of deposit as we approach retirement.

198

With these so-called "safer, risk-free" investments, we can count on a whopping 2-4% annual return that just beats inflation. It's no wonder that many financial advisers want you to have over $1 million in tangible assets. If you're only getting a conservative return of 3%, this equates to a retirement income of $30,000 per year.

There must be a better way. So how do you take back control over your wealth creation? The simple answer - learn how to invest for cash flow, whether it be in the stock market, real estate, systematized businesses or even commodities.

You may be asking yourself: "Now that would require a whole shift in how I've been programmed to think and act." I know that it took me awhile to fully grasp the possibility of a simpler approach to dealing with my lack of retirement capital challenge.

For example (and a simplified one at that), in order to realize an income of $30,000 per year with a 15% return on your capital, you would only need to position $200,000, not a $1 million in the stock and options markets. That's a huge difference! And do-able for most people to realize. It's a far cry from what many in the financial services industry have been saying that you need. Sure, I've given you a simplistic version of what could transpire. But it does illustrate how you could realistically create a cash flowing system with a smaller capital base.

By becoming an active investor, you can continue to build your wealth well into your 70's. As long as you can think clearly, you can profit from being actively involved in generating cash flow from your investments.

This entails building your investments around individual stocks and using simple options strategies to both protect your positions and generate additional cash flow. Much of this section of your book will focus on how you can empower yourself to generate consistent double digit returns through efficient and effective cash flow strategies. Once you have your cash machine in place, you can either systematically tap into the income being generated or allow it to compound over time.

Myth #2: Options trading is too complicated and too risky for the average investor.

True, getting started in options can be daunting. What scares many investors off is the specialized language unique to options trading. As in learning any new skill, the learning curve can be steep.

However, once you have acquired those basic skills, being able to apply that newfound wisdom to increase your ability to make money whether the stock market is going up, down or sideways is well worth the effort. Once you master the special language and start using a few conservative money-making option strategies, you'll wonder why more investors don't do the same thing.

Jay Pestrichelli and ***Wayne Ferbert*** in their book ***Buy and Hedge*** which marries stock investing with options trading say that: *"Hedging your investments changes how you measure risk in your portfolio. It simplifies the process. When you are hedged, you have controlled for your risk."*

Hedging is a term often used to describe the use of either a call or put option to reduce the risk of capital loss, in other words to provide some insurance for your stock holdings. Renting out your stock to other investors - in other words - selling covered calls provides you with both an opportunity to generate additional cash flow as well as cushion your stock from the effects of a temporary drop in the stock price. In effect, options can be used to reduce your overall portfolio risk and make you some additional cash at the same time.

Scott Kyle in his book ***The Power Curve***, in which he advocates smart investing by using dividends, options and the magic of compounding states that: *"Depending on stock and volatility levels, you can often generate 1.5X to 3X in options premium over what is paid in the form of a dividend. For example, if you buy Company X that pays a 5% dividend, you can reasonably generate another 7% to 15% of incremental income annually through the sale of options. During high VIX environments (VIX is a measure of volatility in the markets) the amount of income available from options sales can easily exceed 20% annually."*

Who wouldn't want to learn how to generate returns of 20% just from their options plays?

The top six investment approaches:

To place everything in perspective, let's take a look at six different investment approaches, starting with the most common fixed-income investment - the bond.

Approach #1: Bonds.

Many advisers in the financial services industry advocate placing your money in fixed-income investments such as bonds, especially as you approach retirement.

A typical bond allocation strategy is to set aside a percentage of your overall portfolio for bonds using an age factor. A common calculation is to subtract your age from 110 or 100 to arrive at the percentage of your portfolio that should be in stocks, with the balance in bonds. For example, if you are 50 years old, the formula recommends having between 50-60% of your money in stocks. Therefore, you should have 40-50% of your capital in bonds.

Bonds have traditionally been thought of as being a safe haven compared to stocks, which appear to fluctuate more dramatically in price. But, are bonds really "safer" than stocks?

That depends on what you mean by safer. Successful investing, where you are able to generate consistent inflation-beating returns over the long term, depends on a number of important factors.

One key factor is the effects of inflation. Any investment that is unable to at least keep up with the pace of inflation is risky. You jeopardize the purchase power of your initial capital in the future by not seeking investment vehicles that at least keep up with the rate of inflation as is the case with a savings account that pays much less than the current rate of inflation. Inflation typically rises as long-term interest rates climb.

Bond yields and bond prices have an inverse relationship to each other. When interest rates rise; the price and value of your long-term bonds falls. As well, your bonds get paid back with cheaper dollars due to the effects of inflation thus eroding your purchasing power.

In today's economic climate, long-term bonds with their current low yields of 3 to 4% barely keep up with the rate of inflation. At a 3 percent interest rate, it will take you over 23 years to double your initial investment. That's a lot longer than what most investors are willing to wait nowadays.

Over the long term you will experience an erosion of your purchasing power by being too heavily weighted in any fixed-income investments. Does this sound like a risk-free investment choice to you?

Approach #2: Mutual Funds.

We all want to be able to build our little nest egg over time without a loss of our purchasing power. The stock market has provided the safest opportunity to do so over time, which brings us to the next most common and popular investment vehicle, the mutual fund.

The mutual fund industry has been booming for decades. Billions have been made for both the fund managers and salesmen despite the industry's lack luster performance in comparison to the S&P 500 or DJIA. More than 70 percent of mutual fund managers are unable to consistently beat the broad market indexes such as the S&P 500 over time. Thus, average returns for mutual funds, once you account for fees, have historically been around 5 to 6%, once again just above the rate of inflation.

Unfortunately, many financial advisers will only sell you investments that generate a commission for themselves, and not necessarily the best opportunities for higher returns for you. You'll end up making your advisor rich well before you do. From my point of view that makes as much sense as putting a screen door on a submarine.

The returns of most actively-managed mutual funds fail to keep up with the market averages. When you factor in a Management Expense Ratio (MERs) of 1.5 - 3.5 % of assets per year that all actively-managed mutual funds charge, you significantly reduce your returns over the long term. Also, as the value of the investment rises, the MER represents an increasing dollar amount that is paid out.

Sales charges or "loads" as high as 5% that are paid to the advisor either up front or on the back end further reduce your returns. These numbers are not reflected in the posted returns of mutual funds. With a back-end load fund, in the event that you close your account prior to a specified holding period, which is usually 5 or 6 years long, you're charged back additional percentages for not keeping your money in that fund. This is just another level of risk that you need to account for as a mutual fund investor.

As well, when you buy mutual funds, you're placing the control of your investment decisions in the hands of a fund manager who in all likelihood will underperform the broad market and whose investment approach may fly directly in the face of your desired objectives.

Approach #3: Index Funds.

A better alternative to mutual funds may be the Index Mutual Fund or Exchange Traded Index Fund (ETF) that holds a basket of stocks representing an index such as the S&P 500 or Russell 1000. The index fund attempts to spread the volatility of individual stocks across a huge portion of the market by creating a portfolio of the largest companies in the market. The idea is that by diversifying your holdings across the entire market you reduce your overall risk of having say one stock severely underperforming the others in a small portfolio of 10 holdings.

Since these funds are not actively managed the fees associated with owning them are much less than actively managed mutual funds. Hence, they are able to generate returns that are just below the market averages. These funds have historically generated returns in the range of 7 to 8%.

At this rate of return you could expect to double your portfolio in about 10 years if all goes well and the markets do not experience a couple of major corrections in the same decade as in 2001 and 2008 or the recent minor correction in 2018.

Approach #4: Individual Stocks.

Historically, owning a well-diversified portfolio of individual stocks has generated average returns of 9 to 10%, which is consistent with what you would expect the broad market to experience. This is the arena where the majority of actively-engaged stock investors begin their journey into the wonderful world of stock investing. In the hands of a knowledgeable and experienced investor these returns can creep up into the realm of double-digit returns.

However, without the use of options positions, the stock investor must be very adept in moving into positions when the stocks are undervalued and out of positions when the stocks are overpriced.

The biggest challenge is dealing with strategy risk. One common mistake is where an investor enters a short-term trade position that heads in the wrong direction and rather than cut one's losses the investor simply switches his strategy, which now becomes a long-term buy and "hope it rebounds" position.

Given a historic return of 10%, an actively-engaged investor can expect to double his or her money in about 7 years. Not bad, but can we do better?

Approach #5: Accelerated Cash Flow Approach.

Moving up the food chain of investment options, we arrive at the accelerated cash flow approach to investing, which combines the power of individual stock picks with options positions. A knowledgeable cash flow investor can comfortably generate double digit returns, over long periods of time, in the range of 15 to 20% depending on the strategies employed.

Unfortunately, I can't make you any promises as to what sort of returns you'll generate. Promises are like babies. They're fun to make, but harder to deliver.

The major advantages of combining individual stock picks with options is that you're able to take advantage of the compounding effects of option premiums, and stock appreciation, as well as being able to mitigate your downside risk through the use of strategically placed positions.

The challenge of course is in increasing your financial education to a level where you can profit from a combination of simple yet effective strategies to generate massive cash flow.

The massive appeal of the accelerated cash flow approach to investing is that you're able to rapidly increase your rate of being able to double your holdings, typically within a 4 to 5-year period.

Approach #6: Options Trading.

And last but not least is the world of options trading, which is a double-edged sword. Trading options as a day trader can be very lucrative and rewarding with annual returns upwards of 24%.

However, it has ruined more lives than created wealth because individuals have not taken the time to learn how to effectively trade options and more importantly how to change their mindset to become disciplined, focused and confident traders.

As **Mark Douglas** in his book **Trading in the Zone** so succinctly puts it: *"The goal of any trader is to turn consistent profits on a regular basis, yet so few people ever really make consistent money as traders."*

Why use an Accelerated Cash Flow Investment System?

As you can see, risk comes in many different flavors. You risk losing purchasing power if your investment vehicle is unable to keep up with the rate of inflation, as is the case with most fixed-income investments. You risk being able to generate higher returns because of fees that eat away at your potential capital growth as is the case with mutual funds. You also lose control over how you want to invest and in what investments by turning over the reins to a fund manager. You risk having to wait decades in order to build up any appreciable wealth through index funds. And, you must also resign yourself to amassing a fortune before being able to retire since you have not learned how to generate consistent double-digit returns under various market conditions.

The only risk that faces you now is in committing the time and undertaking the challenge of becoming a cash flow Investor. By taking up this challenge, your odds of becoming wealthy over time increase dramatically. This cash flow investment system is based on two key factors that will accelerate your wealth building process even faster.

Two key wealth building factors to focus on:

Joe Terranova in his book ***Buy High Sell Higher*** says:
"Most investors buy a stock with little thought as to how long they will hold onto it. In addition, few give more than a passing thought to what kind of return they are looking for from any given investment. As a result, they intentionally or unintentionally subscribe to the buy and hold theory of investing, hanging onto assets come hell or high water. Few of us can afford to be like Warren Buffett and hold a stock forever while it dips into negative territory and drags down the rest of our portfolio. Before you invest in any asset, you first need to ask yourself: How long you are willing to tie up your capital with it?"

The critical question that you need to be asking yourself is when do you need to move to another investment opportunity with more strength and momentum that allows you to accelerate your wealth-building? Which brings us to the first key wealth-building factor.

Factor #1: Increasing the Velocity of your money.

Truly successful investors do not park their money and forget about it. They move their money around into better and better opportunities. This is true whether you are talking about stocks, real estate or other business opportunities. This strategy is known as the "velocity of your money."

Your goal in investing should be to acquire cash flowing assets and to continually seek better opportunities that will get you closer to realizing your dreams. The old buy and hold strategy that worked during the last major bull market of 2012 to 2018 no longer works.

As *Joe Terranova* in his book ***Buy High Sell Higher*** states: *"If the buy and hold strategy continued to work one would be able to buy the S&P 500 Index in 2000 and ride the escalator up to higher profits by 2010. That was not the case. The S&P 500 was down roughly 10% in the last decade."*

If such is the case, we need to consider those strategies that'll work in today's markets that have experienced surges in equity and commodity volatility, not to mention the increased uncertainty. In order to accelerate your wealth building process, you have two plans of attack to consider:

The first is to look at how you can increase the velocity of your money within investments. This entails maximizing your profit-making potential by focusing on the combination of option premiums and stock appreciation in your core holdings. Each component adds to your overall return compounding over time to quickly reach a point of critical mass.

The second plan of attack to increase the velocity of your money is between investments. When you get into the habit of monitoring possible opportunities, the odd one could present itself when it meets your specific buy criteria. It is at this point in time that you need to act quickly to move your money in order to take advantage of that window of opportunity.

By creating a winning mindset and planning your investments in advance you increase the chances of moving into these profitable opportunities.

Factor #2: Reaching critical mass.

I briefly mentioned the concept of reaching a point of critical mass with your investments. Let me elaborate. When you start out investing, the compounding effect of your investing slowly builds over time. At a certain point, the compounding effect of your cash flow that you're generating from your investments will exceed your annual household expenses and provide you with your desired lifestyle. It is at this point in time that you have reached a point of critical mass with your investing. This number is different for each and every one of us.

Once you have reached this point of investing prowess, you can now look forward to reaching your financial-freedom day that much sooner. That is my objective - to share with you the wealth of knowledge of the top investment educators currently engaged in the market today through an accelerated cash flow investment system.

Seven things great investors do:

Being on top of your game all the time as a stock market investor has its challenges. What does it take to consistently earn money in the markets today? Here are 7 golden nuggets of wisdom to help get you closer to your investment goals:

Tip #1: Have a positive, "will try hard" attitude all the time. Commit to learning something new about stock investing every day. Be proactive and develop some positive daily learning habits. Set aside some time each morning to stimulate and challenge your mental capacity by reading for fifteen to twenty minutes or listening to an audio book before heading off to work or elsewhere. This tip alone will empower you to be a more consistent and successful investor.

Tip #2: Show a willingness to learn. Be teachable and keep an open mind to learning about the incredible world of investing. You can teach an old dog new tricks. Learning forces you to step out of your "comfort zone" and change the way you think about yourself, others and the wonderful world of investing.

Tip #3: Ask, listen and learn. Use the acronym A.S.K. – Always Seeking Knowledge – to guide you. Let your curiosity take hold of you and move you to another level of understanding about investing by tapping into the wealth of knowledge of those experts who have gone before you. Actively go out and seek answers to your most pressing questions either on blogs, video posts or forums.

Tip #4: Be creative in how you squeeze learning time into your daily routine. Can you combine your exercise time with reading or listening to a personal development tape? How about listening to an audio program while walking the dog or on your morning commute?

Tip #5: Be organized and tidy with your investment information. Keeping your desk area and any investment resource material tidy fosters both increased productivity and greater motivation to stay engaged in learning how to become a better investor. No longer will you get frustrated not knowing where key documents are kept and give up on the whole investment process.

Tip #6: Avoid the time waster of blaming yourself, others or you dog for mistakes you make with your investments. Mistakes ultimately result in an opportunity to learn. Focus on the lessons learned from your failures. Every potential investment presents itself as a unique self-contained opportunity at that particular moment. Keep this in mind for all of your future investment opportunities.

Tip #7: In general, become more of a problem solver. Think of ways to apply what you've just learned. Continuously engage your mind in solving problems or overcoming obstacles in order to achieve greater success. Ask yourself: How could I use this newfound knowledge right now? At the end of each day, reflect on what you've learned and all those little successes you've experienced.

By following these golden nuggets of wisdom, you set yourself up to become a truly great investor.

Investing vs. Trading:

Investor - Trader - Speculator - Gambler. Which one are you?

Scott Kyle in his book ***The Power Curve*** talks about the differences between investing and trading. He points out that: *"Trading is associated with risk-taking and with gambling, but I believe that speculation and gambling are functions not of time frames but mind-sets and one's knowledge basis."*

I tend to concur. It is not the activity that defines whether it is gambling or investing, it is the ability of the educated investor to consistently generate returns that factors in as to whether that activity will be speculative or not.

I think of investing as allocating capital with a time horizon of a year or more with the objective of gaining a return on that money in the form of capital appreciation of the stock price and through cash flow from dividends and options. Trading would be defined as allocating capital with a time frame of less than one year with the goal of generating the same types of returns. It may help to think of your trading and investing opportunities as falling within a time continuum extending from just a few days to several years.

So how does passive vs. active investing fit into this context?

The Passive vs. Active Investor/ Trader:

A passive investor believes that the markets are generally efficient in generating a return on their investment. The passive investor is willing to accept market returns in exchange for little involvement in the process. Most individuals who have their money parked in mutual funds fall into this category. They typically pay hefty management fees to have someone else manage their holdings.

These fees can be substantial and erode your capital appreciation over time. For example, if your mutual fund provides you with an 8% annual return and management fees account for 2%, you're giving up 25% of your potential growth for the convenience of having someone else look after your investments. Not only that, but your broker gets paid no matter what, whether the stocks in the fund go up or down. More about this a bit later in the book.

An active investor believes that the markets are not efficient and that he or she can actively be involved in the process of buying and selling positions thus achieving above average returns. This is the basis of this resource - empowering you to become a better more confident active investor.

Note that you can make money investing, you can make money trading, you can make money being passive, and you can make money being active. These are the choices that every investor has to make at some point in time. When you commit the necessary time to learn how to generate profits in the stock market by actively investing under any market conditions, you'll be light years ahead of the majority of individuals using the traditional buy and pray the stock goes up passive approach.

Kyle goes on to say that:
"While most people think of Warren Buffett as a buy-and-hold only investor, and the typical view of Jim Cramer is that he is a lightning fast trader, these two men are not far apart in terms of style as it would appear. Buffett is constantly getting in and out of positions, be they equities or special situations, from commodities to currencies, to everything in between. Similarly, while Cramer is undoubtedly more active than Buffett in terms of equity holdings, he maintains many positions for years, as long as the fundamentals stay strong. Simply put, the very best money managers are both investors and traders, and they know which hat they are wearing at any point in time and, more importantly, why."

You may hear me using the terms investor and trader interchangeably, since we are both investors and traders depending on the context of the situation. The key is to know in advance whether capital is being allocated for an investment or a trade. You can make money both ways, especially if trading is effectively combined with investing. However, each situation requires a different mindset and approach in order to maximize your potential gains and minimize your risks. Which brings us to ...

The dangers of day trading:

Janet Lowe in her book *The Triumph of Value Investing* cautions investors about the dangers of day trading. She says that: *"There are hundreds of organizations appealing to the gambling instinct in most of us by marketing the idea that you can sit at home all day in your pajamas and earn a fabulous living as a day trader. The pitchmen are making great money providing training, software, and support, which in some cases can cost as much as $45.000."*

Several studies have shown that approximately 70% of day traders lose money and are wiped out within the first year of trading. This book does NOT teach you how to become a day trader.

A fundamental question to keep in the back of your mind as you begin investing is: Am I investing or gambling with my money? Some of the tell-tale signs of individuals who believe that they are investing but actually are gambling are that they:

1. Engage in speculative risk-taking resulting in significant losses in relation to their level of assets.
2. Chase losses through increasing speculation or have difficulty in stopping when they are losing.
3. Borrow excessive amounts of money in order to "invest."
4. Display erratic, inconsistent, or irrational trading behavior.
5. Place trades too frequently.

Follow these 12 pre-defined rules to protect your stock portfolio:

Start by creating a system of rules that define specifically at what point you'll both exit and enter an opportunity based on likely outcomes or probabilities. Then, stick to those rules when an investment triggers a course of action to take as the market moves either in one direction or another.

Here are the top 12 basic rules that many of the investment industry's respected experts suggest that you consider as part of your overall investment plan:

1. Own the best of breed; it's worth it. When the choice is among two or three companies in an industry, always go for the industry leader regardless of the price.

2. If you want to build a sizeable position over time, buy in increments. Don't buy all at once. Always keep a small portion of your regular contributions in cash for those market breaks.

3. It is impossible to own more than 20 stocks unless you are a full-time stock junkie. The right-sized diversified portfolio where you can do it yourself is between 5 and 10 stocks.

4. Sitting in cash on the sidelines may be a fine alternative. When the market is overvalued, take stock off, raise cash and get ready for the next decline. Sell strength and buy weakness in the stocks of companies you love and understand.

5. Buy stocks that you believe should go higher because of the fundamentals and avoid stocks where the underlying business is bad or getting worse. Also, monitor those companies that have unfairly been beaten up despite solid fundamentals. They may provide great growth opportunities.

6. Take your profits off the table. Keep in mind that you don't have a profit until you sell. You should not confuse book gains with real gains. Those gains not taken can turn out to be losses down the road. Always take profits rather than worry about paying taxes and losing out on an opportunity entirely.

7. Take excessive emotional mood swings out of investing. Stick to your process of investing. A patient, less panicked style of investing always generates a higher return.

8. Be flexible and open to change. Something good one month can turn bad. Stay on top of monitoring each position.

9. Just because someone says it on TV doesn't make it so. Don't trust anything you hear. Do your own due diligence. If you like it and understand it, then buy it.

10. Cut your losses quickly. It's okay to take a loss when you already have one. A loss is a loss whether realized or unrealized. By controlling your losses, you can let your winners do the running.

11. Don't buy or sell stock on any tip. All of your trades require that you do your due diligence to verify if the opportunity merits action on your part. Remember, tips are for waiters, not for traders.

12. Be patient. Sometimes a stock on your watch list that you like does nothing for ages. Many turnarounds take 12 - 18 months before the business takes off. Eventually, these stocks, especially if they are undervalued, rise up to their true intrinsic value.

Top 5 pitfalls to investing and trading:

The following are the top five pitfalls to investing that set back many a novice investor according to some of the top investment educators in the market today:

Pitfall #1: Ignoring the learning curve.

It is critical to your long-term success as an investor to work on your weaknesses while playing to your strengths. It takes time to develop an investor-trader mindset that'll serve you well in any type of market environment. With patience and perseverance, you'll eventually achieve your core desires that are motivating you to become a cash flow investor. Take the time to gain the knowledge first, then the experience. As well, learn from your mistakes don't just dismiss them without analyzing the why behind the error.

Pitfall #2: Lacking formal training.

Robert Kiyosaki in his book **Rich Dad's Guide to Investing** says that if you think of time as being precious and that it has a price, the richer you'll become. The poor measure in money and the rich measure in time. If you desire to be rich you need to invest in something more valuable than money, time in learning and studying about investment.

As you learn new skills your financial IQ increases. By taking the time to learn how to use multiple strategies in building your wealth, you quickly build your confidence, which will serve you well for decades down the road. How much better would that be? Focus on becoming a consummate learner and keep an open mind to learning new concepts and approaches.

Pitfall #3: Expecting radical success and huge profits too soon.

Unfortunately, the internet is full of get rich quick schemes that promise riches beyond your wildest dreams in unrealistic time frames and with incredible risk to your hard-earned capital.

With any initial venture, it's important to set realistic expectations and look for smaller returns to start. By keeping your goals modest in the beginning and taking baby steps, your ability to succeed over time increases dramatically. Start by putting in your time learning and gaining experience. The market is going nowhere. There will always be great opportunities for you to realize significant profits over time.

Pitfall #4: Overtrading and risking too much.

Your primary objective has to be to preserve your precious capital. This means that you cannot afford to take on too much risk or chase the market for higher returns. This pitfall often stems from a lack of patience with your progress. The stark reality is that it will require effort on your part to change who you are as an investor so that you can effortlessly move into and out of opportunities without increased risk or over exposure. As well, we all learn at different rates. There is no point in trying to rush the transformational process at the expense of your capital.

Pitfall #5: Lack of consistency and increased frustration.

Investing is simply a plan and a system, made up of formulas and strategies that allow you to become wealthy. If a formula is overly complex, it's not worth following. If you're following too many strategies at once, you'll probably abandon your efforts out of sheer frustration.

Consistent Investing involves these 3 steps:
1. *Preparation* - which is doing your research and due diligence on every investment opportunity.
2. *Planning* - what approach and strategies you'll use to enter and exit your positions.
3. **Pre-commitment** - to a specific investment strategy when in a rational state of mind.

Keep in mind that optimism or hope is not a good investment strategy. You need to plan in advance how you'll anticipate entering and exiting your positions so that you can optimize your returns.

Chapter 10: How Do I Become a Do-It-Yourself Investor?

Now that you have a better understanding as to how you could proceed, let's get you set up with the appropriate investment accounts.

The actual process of setting up these accounts is a simple one. It's a matter of contacting an online discount broker and following their account set-up procedures.

Making the best of your 401(k) & IRA:

Two of the most common investment accounts for retirement are the 401(K) and the IRA. Knowing which account to use in various investment situations can be tricky. Here are some simple investment account tips that might point you in the right direction to maximize your returns and minimize your future tax burden.

There are several main advantages in contributing to a 401(K).
1. You can deposit a lot of money each year compared to other plans.
2. Your employer can match funds that you deposit up to a set maximum.
3. Nobody can touch the money, even if you go bankrupt.
4. Most employers allow you to borrow your own money, paying back the loan over time.
5. Contributions come from pre-tax income, so you don't get taxed on the money going in.

The downside is that:
1. Most plans are very limited in the investment choices that you have. You're typically limited to a few mutual funds and bonds.
2. The average 401(K) fees are 1.5 percent off the top every year. This small amount ends up reducing your potential gains by 40 - 60 percent over time. Yes, you heard me right, your potential returns will be eroded by 40 to 60 percent depending on the time frame selected. This is one major reason why you can do better on your own with a self-directed investment account.

So how do we maximize our profitability in our 401(K) accounts?

If your employer is matching your contributions, then you should contribute money to your plan up to the set maximum for matching funds.

If your company offers a Roth 401(k), then your best bet may be to opt in for this plan as it allows you make withdrawals after age 59 ½ tax free, as opposed to being tax deferred. Having tax-free income in retirement is a great option to have whether or not tax rates will change in the future. My personal feeling is that tax rates will probably increase in the future as opposed to decrease. Of course, the main disadvantage is that the contributions come out of your paycheck after taxes have been removed.

In either 401(k) plans, choose either a low-cost Index Fund that mirrors a broad index like the S&P 500 or possibly get some bond exposure by buying specific bonds. Avoid actively managed mutual funds, since the management fees will erode your profit potential substantially over time.

Avoid both target-date retirement funds and bond funds. Target-date funds create a blend of stock and bond funds based on your retirement date, with a higher allocation to bond funds as you approach retirement. The problem is that long-term bond funds have no set maturity date; therefore, you have less of a guarantee that you'll get your principal back as with individual bonds. This is just one risk factor that you need to be aware of when working with funds.

After you have maxed out your 401(K) matching contributions, the next strategy is to make contributions to an Individual Retirement Account (IRA). An IRA provides you with several key advantages, namely:
1. You have greater flexibility as to what investments you can hold within your account, especially with individual stocks.
2. It allows almost anyone who has earned income to invest.
3. The contributions to a Traditional IRA come from pre-tax income, so under most conditions you don't get taxed on the money going in.
4. Most IRA accounts allow you to sell covered calls, which provides you with a powerful investment platform from which to implement the accelerated cash flow system.

5. Given the choice of different types of IRA accounts, consider opening up a Roth IRA instead of a traditional one. The two major advantages of using a Roth IRA are that:
6. The earnings are tax-free instead of tax-deferred. As already mentioned, this can be significant 10, 20 or even 30 years down the road.
7. You can take out your original contributions any time you want, regardless of your age, without taxes and penalties.

In a nutshell, we're all born free and then you're taxed to death. So, it makes sense to structure your investment portfolios to reduce the effects of taxation on your holdings.

You'll need to set up an account with an online discount broker if you haven't done so already. Start by doing a little comparative research online. This should yield a couple of promising discount brokers who offer low stock and option transaction fees. Select a solid broker who does offer low fees. Higher fees can erode your cash flow potential over time. As the martial arts master says to his young accolade: "Choose wisely Grasshopper."

It's in your IRA account that you'll benefit the most from building a portfolio of stocks, especially if the capital appreciation is able to grow tax-free until you need it in retirement. All discount brokers will allow you to sell calls from within your IRA, which is a key component of the accelerated cash flow system. Please contact your specific online broker to find out what you can and cannot do within your IRA account. Guidelines change from time to time. There you have it in a nutshell, a few simple strategies to incorporate into your overall investment plan.

Are You Canadian, eh?

Making the best of your RRSP & TFSA:

The most common Canadian investment account for retirement is the Registered Retirement Savings Plan or RRSP. However, another savings program that has gained in popularity is the Tax-Free Savings Account. Here are some simple investment account tips that'll give you greater insight into how to use each type of account. There are several main advantages in contributing to a RRSP:

1. You can contribute a high percentage of earned income each year based on the lower of 18% of earned income or a fixed cap, which has been indexed to be slightly over $26,000.
2. You receive a tax credit that reduces your taxable income by the amount you contribute.
3. You are able to defer paying any tax until funds are withdrawn, which is normally at retirement thus allowing your returns to compound tax free over time.
4. You can borrow funds from your account to purchase a home or pay for post-secondary education.
5. You have the flexibility of holding many different types of investments within the account.
6. You can swap investments between another investment portfolio and your RRSP account.
7. You don't lose your contribution room. Any unused contributions are carried forward to your future deduction limits until age 71.

The downside of an RRSP is that:
1. There is a lack of liquidity should you need to use your funds. The tax consequences for early withdrawals can be serious with withholding taxes in the range of 10 to 30%, in addition to your income tax payable.
2. You can't take advantage of the dividend tax credit on eligible shares that are part of an RRSP. As well, the full amount of capital gains realized within a RRSP is eventually fully taxable at retirement or withdrawal. Capital gains that are not part of an RRSP are subject to income tax on only 50% of the gain, excluding your tax-free savings account. The bottom line? This means that any growth in your RRSP will be eventually taxed at the highest level, that of earned income.

So how do we maximize your profitability potential in your RRSP account?

Your first order of business is to select the right RRSP account. You have two basic choices: a "managed" account, which is usually offered by major financial institutions and mutual fund companies or a "self-directed" account, typically offered by discount brokers.

A managed account limits your investment options to primarily two types of investments, namely mutual fund products and fixed-income investments such as guaranteed investment certificates or GICs.

By choosing a self-directed RRSP you open up your investment possibilities to being able to use the cash flow strategies outlined in this program. For example, from within a self-directed RRSP you'll be able to invest in individual stocks and covered call contracts. Your best bet is to set up your self-directed account with a discount broker thus allowing you access to not only a myriad of investment choices but also low transaction fees that will help to keep your costs down.

Optimizing Your Tax-Free Savings Account:

Most investors are unaware of the growth potential that a simple tax-free savings account can offer a savvy investor. Many use the account as a simple savings program rather than using it to their full advantage. Properly structured, a TFSA can be used to hold quality dividend-paying stocks, or any market leading stock for that matter, and even allow you to sell covered calls. We'll get into options strategies more in the next chapter.

Suffice it to say that the beauty of the TFSA is that any growth is tax exempt, which means that you can use the power of compounding from within the account to accelerate your wealth building even faster.

The account is very liquid, allowing you the flexibility to make withdrawals without penalty. The one limiting factor is that you'll need to wait until January of the following year in order to make any additional contributions up to your allowable limit. The best part is that when you withdraw your funds you won't have to pay any income tax on the withdrawal.

The two biggest limitations of the TFSA are that:
1. The maximum annual contribution limit is currently $5500 (2018) per person.
2. Any contributions made are done so with money that has already been taxed.

So how can we take advantage of the benefits of these various types of accounts? I believe that every Canadian should try to capitalize on the advantages offered by each account.

The TFSA allows you to slowly build a portfolio of stock holdings over time since you're only allowed to contribute $5,500 per year. The biggest advantage is that any gains made in your account are tax free. That will be a huge advantage down the road as you approach retirement.

Your self-directed RRSP also offers great flexibility in terms of being able to use the various cash flow strategies outlined in this program. It allows you to buy quality dividend-paying stocks and then sell monthly covered calls in order to generate a cash flow stream from both the quarterly dividend payments and the monthly option premiums. This account makes sense for someone wanting to compound their gains over time.

The third type of account that unfortunately receives no preferential tax treatment is an option account set up with your discount broker. This account gives you the greatest flexibility of investment strategies to employ. You'll also be able to take advantage of the 50% exclusion rule on capital gains and the dividend tax credit on eligible dividends. Eligible dividends are those paid by Canadian companies to Canadian tax payers; therefore, foreign companies such as Intel or McDonalds are unfortunately exempt.

At a bare minimum, an accelerated cash flow investor should open up a self-directed RRSP and TFSA that allows stock and option plays. To get a better feel for what each account has to offer and what the rules, regulations and tax implications are for each account, go to the Revenue Canada website.

Three stock investment approaches:

A simplistic view of how you can invest in the stock market is to look at three current practices used extensively by most investors. These three approaches are value, income and growth investing.

Each approach provides the investor with different investment opportunities offering:
1. Different risk - reward profiles.
2. Varying investment holding periods.
3. And the use of various stock investment strategies.

The following is a simplified explanation of these common approaches.

Value Investing:

The primary objective of value investing is to acquire undervalued businesses below fair market price and hold them long-term until they can be sold above their true intrinsic value at a profit.

The key factors of value investing are that:
1. The primary focus is on capital preservation by buying the business with a large margin of safety below its fair market price. A margin of safety refers to a current stock price that is typically 30% or more less than the stock's estimated intrinsic value or retail price.
2. Select businesses with solid fundamentals in the areas of book value, debt levels, and return on capital invested over a minimum 5-year period.
3. The holding period is long-term, typically 5 - 10 years.
4. The type of investor favored is one with a low risk tolerance and who is patient and disciplined.
5. You profit best from the stock price cycling from being undervalued to overvalued.

Income Investing:

The objective of income investing is to create a regular, income stream from typically mature companies who consistently pay a portion of profits back to the shareholders in the form of dividends.
The key factors of income investing are that:
1. The primary focus is on regular income production, at least quarterly, with an emphasis on capital preservation by investing in companies that have a long solid track record.

2. Select mature businesses with consistent earnings, sales and cash flow over long periods of 10 to 20 years that have a historical record of paying good dividends.
3. The holding period is usually long-term, typically greater than 10 years.
4. The type of investor favored is one with a low risk tolerance, who is typically looking for income generation, such as in retirement or helping to fund a college education.
5. You profit best from mature businesses that are not greatly affected by economic cycles and who have a solid track record of consistently paying out dividends.

Growth Investing:

The primary objective of growth investing is to acquire businesses experiencing higher than market average earnings growth due to a major change affecting the industry. Ideally, the investor would like to select businesses in their infancy of their growth phase. They have the greatest potential to grow and become more stable mature companies down the road.

The key factors of growth investing are that:
1. The primary focus is on capital appreciation through increased share price in companies experiencing a major positive change in their industry. This typically happens as a result of new technological breakthroughs, new market trends or expanding international markets.
2. Select specialized businesses or industries experiencing positive change and that have superior growth in earnings, sales and a strong possibility of high growth of invested capital.
3. The holding period is often medium-term, typically 2 - 5 years.
4. The type of investor favored is one with a moderate risk tolerance who is typically looking for capital appreciation.
5. You profit best from younger companies that are seeing the benefits from a major market change that is enabling them to grow earnings and invested capital above the market average.

All three approaches have their place in an investor's portfolio, whether you're just starting out or you're at the end of your pursuit as an active investor. Having said that, the question that begs to be answered is so how does an accelerated cash flow system differ from the above general investment approaches?

How does an Accelerated Cash Flow System fit in?

In a nutshell, an accelerated cash flow system is based on an income and growth approach that incorporates option strategies to generate higher returns than any one approach on its own.

The basic premise behind being able to accelerate your returns is that you'll build a portfolio of core growth positions. Ideally, we're looking for growing companies that are market leaders and best of breed in their respective market sector or industry.

A market leader has the general market and price momentum behind it. Many big institutional buyers look for stocks within a specific sector or industry that the overall market has fallen in love with. These stocks are in favour as evidenced by a positive growing trend in world demand for the products or services being offered.

For example, in 2011 and 2012 the mobile internet was one growing trend worldwide that had many technology stocks moving higher as a result of being in favour with the overall market players. And currently many cannabis-related stocks are showing appreciable gains especially with Canada legalizing marijuana as of October 17, 2018.

The companies that are market leaders are those that are benefiting the most from the sale of their products and services in the worldwide market. They also tend to be the best of breed businesses within their industry. A best of breed business is one that has:
1. *Solid fundamentals.*
This shows up in the key ratios that are showing consistent double-digit growth rates and long-term debt levels that are under control.

2. A solid management team.
Here we're looking for a CEO who comes across as having his/her shareholder's interest at heart and not his/her ego or the bonuses he/she might receive.

3. A competitive advantage.
Having a sustainable competitive advantage sets any business apart from other companies that are just along for the ride in a trending market. Determining if a company has a significant competitive advantage is easily verified by looking at the growth rates for earnings, sales, cash flow and book value. More on that in a moment, okay?

Best of breed businesses have the staying power to be profitable over time, which in turn increases your profitability potential as an investor. We'll take a look at how to spot these businesses in the next chapter. An accelerated cash flow approach focuses on using the momentum of the stock market to build wealth. As previously mentioned, it is based on two wealth building factors.

The first is increasing the velocity of your money by accelerating your cash flow coming from your stock holdings. This is not a buy, hold and pray strategy. Your investment dollars will move from one great business to even better ones over the course of the year. By having your investment capital generating monthly cash flow that can be re-invested into additional opportunities should you choose, you're able to create a constant stream of income flowing into your brokerage account.

As **Jim Cramer** puts it in his book **Getting Back to Even**:
"Most peddlers of financial advice, even after the wealth-shattering crash of 2008, preach the virtues of owning stock just for the sake of owning them. They will tell you to buy and hold, an investing shibboleth that I have been trying to smash for ages. The buy-and-hold strategy, if you can even call it one, is to pick a bunch of good-looking blue-chip companies, buy their stocks, and hang on to them till kingdom come. Selling is strictly forbidden. It's considered a sign of recklessness, of "trading," which all too many supposed experts think of as a dirty word. Same goes for the once-sacred mutual funds, with mangers who adopted the same careless buy-and-hold, one-decision philosophy."

225

The second factor is reaching a point of critical mass with your investments. Critical mass is achieved when the cash flow from your investments equals or exceeds your expenses for your desired lifestyle. This is a primary objective of this book. Enable you to generate enough cash flow so that you can live the life of your dreams and provide for your family without worry.

Why covered calls?

Selling covered calls has some great benefits, such as:
Benefit #1: Tap into additional monthly or bi-monthly income.
You can generate a nice stream of additional income from selling option contracts on stock that you already own. This strategy alone can generate double-digit returns for your portfolio over the course of a year.

Selling a covered call is a conservative option strategy. **Michael Thomsett** in his book **Options Trading for the Conservative Investor** says that: *"The properly selected covered call strategy produces consistent current income. In exchange for writing covered calls, you risk losing out on an increased market value; when stock prices rise above strike price and calls are exercised, your shares are called away. However, when you compare that risk to the regular and dependable creation of current income in a conservative market risk profile, it is apparent that covered call writing will beat market averages without increasing market risks."*

I know that was a mouthful. In a nutshell **Thomsett** touts the virtues of selling covered calls as a conservative income producing strategy in the stock market.

Benefit #2: Reduces risk.
Since you're paid a premium for renting out your stock, that cash now reduces your initial cost price or basis for the stock. Your breakeven point, should the stock decline in price, has been lowered by the amount of the premium deposited directly into your brokerage account.

In essence, you've built in a margin of safety for preserving your initial capital. Over time as you continue to write covered calls, which is another way of saying selling covered calls, your cost basis of the stock will drop to zero.

Now we're generating a cash flow from an initial investment whereby you've recovered all of your initial capital even with a stock that may not have appreciated in stock price. You're in the enviable position of playing with the house's money, as they say in Vegas. Wouldn't that be cool?

Benefit #3: Accelerates your wealth creation.
When you're able to generate a cash flow from multiple sources, such as options and dividends, this accelerates the velocity of your money in moving your capital into better and better investments. Being able to generate cash from various sources also allows you to have access to capital for opportunities when they present themselves. And did we mention the compounding effect earlier? Re-investing your proceeds gets you that much closer to reaching your point of critical mass with your investment portfolio.

As a novice options trader, there is no reason to start out learning complex strategies. Some of the simplest most conservative strategies can be the most lucrative.

One of my favorite conservative option trading strategies allows me to generate a monthly or bi-monthly income from my stock holdings. But before I share this simple strategy with you, we need to take a look at the concept of options trading.

What are options?

There are only two types of options - a call and a put - that can be either bought or sold. All option trading strategies are based on only these four factors. We'll be focusing our attention on just selling calls in this particular book.

By using a very conservative call option strategy that of selling covered calls, you can create some additional monthly income. This strategy works well when the markets are slowing trending upward (what is known as a bullish trend) or the markets are going nowhere - being essentially flat month to month.

The call option strategy of selling covered calls is simple to implement. The basic idea is to "rent out" your shares of stock on a monthly or bi-monthly basis, in which you're paid a premium up front (the rent) in doing so. To rent out your shares, you must own at least 100 shares of stock for every option contract that you sell. Following me so far?

When you sell your contract, the buyer on the other end of the transaction now has the right to buy your stock at a specified fixed price, known as the strike price. The buyer can do so only when the stock price is at or above the strike price by a specific date known as the expiration date. The buyer can then choose to buy your stock at any time before this expiration date once it is at or above the strike price.

You may be saying to yourself, hold on there R.J., that sounds like a losing proposition. Why would I want to rent out my stock only to see it being sold down the road? I thought that I was investing in the stock market to create wealth, not to be kicked out onto the sidelines.

Even if your stock is called away, that is sold at or prior to expiration, at your agreed upon strike price, you still can profit from the situation. Suffice it to say, that in an upcoming section, you'll learn how to properly structure each covered call position so that you can optimize your profitability when we discuss various strategies in greater detail.

If you had set your strike price above your initial price paid for the stock you not only get to keep the premium from selling the call option, but you have also captured the capital gain of the stock rising from its initial price to the strike price. As well, you're positioned to take advantage of the next opportunity that presents itself.

I have found myself being exercised, that is to say having my stock called away, on a couple of occasions with the cannabis stocks that I owned. Not only did I pick up both the call option premium and the capital gain on the stock price appreciation, within a week later I bought back into the same stock at a lower price point than my initial purchase price. Not a bad scenario at all. Just rinse and repeat when the opportunity presents itself. Could you see yourself benefiting from a similar scenario?

When you learn how to control your cash flow that is being generated from your options plays, you'll see the full potential behind selling covered calls.

Chapter 11: Where Do I Find Wonderful Stocks?

Using a top-down approach:

Every stock investor would love to own a portfolio of stocks that has the greatest potential for consistent capital appreciation over time with limited downside risk. The challenge is in knowing which stocks to place on your watch list of top candidates. Here's one stock selection strategy to help you with the decision-making process.

By looking initially at what the overall economy is doing, you can narrow down those sectors or industries that offer the best growth prospects over the next couple of years. Why just a few years? The harsh reality is that the economy expands and contracts on average every 4 to 6 years. So, trying to make realistic growth projections for time periods greater than 2-3 years becomes extremely challenging for any investor.

A short-term top-down approach takes a macro (or bird's eye) view of the economy. Imagine being a forester who focuses on looking at the health of the overall forest before checking out the individual trees that can be harvested. Your initial goal is to place more emphasis on identifying market trends that will support certain sectors and then select those industries that will benefit from the trends. Once you have a feel for the overall market, you can drill down and select the best businesses in each industry or sector. Good, so far?

Here are three questions that help me get started in assessing the current market environment:

Question #1: *Is the economy expanding, contracting or experiencing a recession?*
This information is readily available from government sources, as well as from several major financial websites like Yahoo Finance, MSN Money or Morningstar. Look for official announcements indicating the state of affairs of the economy.

Question #2: What is the primary trend in the stock market?
By looking at a technical chart of a broad index such as the S&P 500 you can assess whether or not recent market conditions have been neutral (as in 2011), bullish (a positive outlook) or bearish (a negative outlook).

Question #3: What is the interest rate trend?
If interest rates are rising there may be competition from high-quality fixed-income instruments (like bonds) that may impact how money flows into and out of the stock market. More importantly, higher interest rates affect economic sectors differently.

Businesses listed on the major stock market exchanges can be loosely grouped into 11 economic sectors of like businesses representing key areas of the economy. Examples of some specific observations that you can use to your advantage in screening for a promising economic sector of stocks are:

1. A low inflation rate trend will benefit the retailing industry.
2. A high inflation rate trend benefits the mining sector.
3. A slowdown in consumer spending affects the consumer staples sector the least.
4. A strengthening economy benefits the consumer discretionary sector which tends to be cyclical in nature.
5. A slowing economy is beneficial for health care and consumer staples, which are known as defensive stocks in a bad economy.
6. Rapidly increasing global debt has a negative impact on the financial sector.

Once you have identified in which sectors to concentrate your efforts, you can then start screening for those top-notch businesses that are the market leaders in their respective industries.

Seven megatrends to keep your eye on:

In keeping in line with our top-down approach, here are seven global trends that could provide you with some potential stock investing opportunities related to the cannabis industry.

Trend #1: Edibles.

Not everyone wants to or is capable of smoking marijuana. This is where edible products fill the void. As bakers and candy makers develop their skills in creating pastries, cookies, bars, and candy treats, so does the potential for businesses to take off. Look for regional chains that may be taking their business to a national level as the demand for cannabis-based food products increases.

Trend #2: Beverage Industry.

Constellation Brands has already made a substantial investment in the cannabis industry by partnering with Canopy Growth (WEED). Being one of the largest international alcoholic beverage conglomerates in the World, they have already positioned themselves to take advantage of the exponential growth in the industry. Where cannabis consumption is already legal winemakers and brew masters are already experimenting with cannabis-infused alcoholic beverages. Energy and soft drink producers are also looking at ways to incorporate cannabis into their products. Coca-Cola was in talks with Aurora Cannabis (ACB) to do just that.

Trend #3: Pharmaceutical Industry.

The over 50 crowd is the fastest growing sector of the American population. As this segment of the population ages they will require more services related to health care. Pharmaceutical companies and drug retailers should see steadily increasing demand for their products, even should a recession hit. The growth potential of the cannabis industry as more and more jurisdictions worldwide move to legalizing marijuana, will eventually filter into big pharma.

Trend #4: Food Processing Industry.

Marijuana once harvested needs to be processed before it can be used for anything other than smoking and vaping. This is where the food and medical processing industries step in. They provide the high-tech processing that enables the bud to be purified and converted into a form that the food and beverage industries use. In fact, in those states where the recreational use of cannabis is legal, fewer individuals are choosing to purchase buds for smoking and more of the general public is buying cannabis products made primarily from refined oils. Businesses that produce cannabis extracts will do extremely well in the future.

Trend #5: Pet Care.

The market for pet therapeutics is growing as more jurisdictions loosen their marijuana laws. If cannabis has health benefits for humans, could it also be beneficial in certain cases for our furry four-legged friends? You betcha. The American Veterinary Association has called for roadblocks on research be lifted. Over time we'll see more business opportunities evolve as a direct result of this growing trend. Cannabis pet care products could even surpass the traditional marijuana market in sales.

Trend #6: Bio Diesel from Hemp.

As technology advances so does the feasibility of bringing bio diesel products to market. Bio diesel made from plant-based material is a renewable energy source. Many nations are exploring ways to decrease their dependence on crude oil by leaning towards other alternative sources of power. Bio diesel made from hemp is one such alternative. Once jurisdictions move to abolish outdated laws limiting the production of hemp, this'll open up the door for entrepreneurs to create new ways of generating energy. Taken to the next level, we could be seeing lucrative businesses producing bio diesel made from hemp on a national scale.

Trend #7: Building Materials from Hemp.

Two of the largest consumers of building materials are China and India whose economies will continue to grow over the next decade. Companies that should see a steady growth in sales as a result of increasing demand for construction material are those producing materials used in construction. Unlike wood, which requires 40+ years between harvests, hemp can be grown annually. It also has physical properties that make it a better product than wood in some applications. This industry may be a few years away from being a major international player. However, once it does become established, you'll see some great stock investment opportunities unfold.

There you have it - seven trends in the cannabis industry that could provide you with some awesome investment opportunities down the road. As a side note, when researching online for potential stock picks, look for those that also trade in the options market. These stocks typically have established themselves enough to be viable choices when you're looking to invest. You'll eventually want to be able to generate additional income and protect your initial investment through the use of covered calls. More on that in a moment, alright?

Four great sources of information to help you find potential stocks:

Here are 4 tips that'll save you some time conducting your initial research in discovering those profitable best-of-breed businesses that can move you closer to reaching your point of financial freedom.

Tip #1: Check Out Free Websites.
Stock screening tools are available on several free websites such as Yahoo Finance and MSN Money. Using the search capabilities of each site you can find potential industries that might be of interest and then drill down to come up with a list of businesses that should have meaning to you.

Tip #2: National Business News Channels.

Look for potential stock picks on business news channels like CNBC, PBS or your favorite national business news station. Sometimes you can get great leads on businesses to consider in your initial investigation by watching financial news programs. Jot down the names of those potential companies that tweak your interest. Something to consider, right?

Tip #3: The Print Media.

The 3rd great source is through the print media. Books, magazines and newspapers are another source of potential companies to explore. Before buying any book or magazine or thinking about subscribing to any newspaper, save yourself some money by checking out the various sources at your local library.

There are a multitude of magazines to choose from, such as Forbes, Fortune, Smart Money and Smart Investor. As far as newspapers, check out the Wall Street Journal or The New York Times for ideas.

Tip #4: Stock Investment Websites.

What words of wisdom could you gleam from various stock investment blogs and websites? There's a lot of free information available on the web.

You can also check out paid subscription sites such as the Blue Collar Investor, American Association of Independent Investors, Motley Fool's Stock Advisor, The Street.com or Investor's Business Daily for suggestions.

Now that you have a better idea as to how to find potential candidates, let's narrow down your watch list by looking at assessing the growth potential of each prospect. To do so, I'll share some basic selection criteria to help you assess the viability of your picks.

The identification and assessment of potential stocks can be a tedious process. Wherever possible, the smart cash flow investor will use those free or inexpensive tools that make the selection process faster and easier.

The extent of research and effort that you'll put in boils down to three factors:

1. How much time you have to realistically do your due diligence.
2. Whether or not your stock will be held long-term as an investment, or short-term as a cash flow trade as in the case of a monthly covered call.
3. Your personal preference as to how much money you could allocate to tap into the speed and convenience offered by subscription sites like The Blue Collar Investor.

My advice to every upcoming investor is to initially learn how to use the assessment criteria as part of your overall selection process. Once you understand how each particular factor helps you identify those best-of-breed industry leaders that offer you the greatest upside potential, then you can begin to streamline your selection process as you become more familiar with what each factor has to offer. Does that make sense?

I can also offer these words of wisdom that may help guide you in your decision-making process:

1. The longer your holding period for your stock pick the more effort you should put into the assessment process. For example, if you are looking for a quality dividend-paying stock that you would like to hang onto for at least one year, then take the time to check out the business thoroughly.
2. The greater the reward and risk involved in the selection of a particular investment strategy the more time you should spend assessing the upside potential of the stock you're considering.

Let's take a look at some of the personal favorite assessment criteria used by many of the successful stock investors and educators in today's marketplace.

Top 9 assessment criteria for Best of Breed businesses:

You may have noticed that when you screened for a particular type of stock several criteria were used in the selection process for finding great stocks. This is critical to identifying fundamentally sound businesses with upside growth potential.

According to **James O'Shaughnessy** in his book **What Works on Wall Street: The Classic Guide to the Best-Performing Investment Strategies of All Time**:

"using several value factors together in a composited value factor offers much better and more consistent returns than using individual value factors on their own." What O'Shaughnessy is saying is that a multi-variable screening approach provides the investor with a higher quality list of potential best-of-breed businesses from which to choose.

Let me jump right in with a list of the top 9 indicators that I like to use for both finding great stocks and assessing their potential. This list is by no means an exhaustive or exclusive list. It has served me and other cash flow investors well in identifying market leaders who are top-notch businesses. I've based my list on what several of the top investment experts have used in their selection process. By looking at recent best practices in the stock investment industry, I was able to drill down and create a short list of the most popular criteria for finding wonderful businesses for your stock portfolio.

Without further ado, here are the top 9 indicators that many of the top dogs like to use for finding great stocks:

1. Return on invested capital (ROIC) being greater than 10%.
2. Book value per share growth rate (BVPS) of at least 10%.
3. Earnings per share growth rate (EPS) being greater than 10%.
4. Revenue or sales growth rate greater than 10%.
5. Cash flow growth rate of 10%.
6. Debt-to-equity ratio (D/E) which should be low and preferably less than 0.5.
7. Price-to-earning-to-growth ratio (PEG) of less than 1.0.
8. Price-to-sales ratio (P/S) which should be low, preferably under 1.0.
9. Relative strength index (RSI) should be high for momentum plays within a range of 60 to 80.

All of the "growth rates" mentioned above should be consistent over a minimum 5-year period. In general, what I look for is consistent growth in earnings over a period of 5 to 7 years and with the capital being generated being put to good use by the management to grow the business.

Yes. I realize that many cannabis companies don't have a 5-year track record for sales and revenue growth. Many of these players just recently listed themselves on the stock market. This makes it challenging trying to figure out whether a company will be profitable moving forward. To quote the great Elmer Fudd: "Be vewy, vewy careful."

Look to those companies that are looking at partnering with some of these up-coming cannabis companies. Investing in these well-established stocks may be the ticket, as new markets open up. Choose stocks in well-established industries like the food and beverage industry for potential picks. If you can't invest directly in a cannabis company at least you can be a part of a growing industry by aligning yourself with those companies that have an underlying agreement to do future business together.

Now that you have an idea as to which factors you can use in your assessment process let's take a look at how each of these 9 factors can be used in our assessment process.

Five key growth rates:

A common question that I am asked is: Which financial numbers do I need to listen to in order to confirm the strength of a business?

Ideally, you want to be able to use just a handful of indicators that help you determine whether you can both trust and predict that the business can deliver double-digit returns in the future. We want to keep the process as simple as possible. We also want to be able to compare rates of change as opposed to the raw numbers. Monitoring rates of change goes hand-in-hand with the concept of increasing the velocity of your money. Some of the most popular indicators and the top five that I personally use in my assessment process are:

Factor #1: Return on Investment Capital (ROIC).

The ROIC is the rate of return a business makes on the cash it invests every year. The ROIC is a measure of how effective a company uses its own and borrowed money invested in its operations. I place greater weight on this fundamental ratio as it tells the investor how effective the business is in using invested capital. This ratio is a strong predictor that the business has a competitive advantage in its industry.

Factor #2: Equity or Book Value per Share Growth Rate (BVPS).

The BVPS is what a business would be worth if it's no longer a business. This would be the liquidation value or book value of the company. The raw number is not important since factory-type businesses can vary immensely with intellectual property businesses. It's the rate of equity growth that is key in comparing businesses. We're looking for businesses that are able to accumulate a growing surplus over time and not spending excessive funds to build new capital-intensive projects.

Factor #3: Earnings per Share Growth Rate.

The EPS indicates how much the business is profiting per share of ownership. The EPS is often found as the last line on the income statement. However, we're more concerned with the growth rate, which we'll either quickly calculate on our own or find in certain financial websites reporting on business fundamentals.

Factor #4: Sales or Revenue Growth Rate.

The sales growth rate represents the total dollars the business took in from selling its products and services. It's usually located on the top line of the income statement.

Factor #5: Free Cash Flow Growth Rate.

Free cash flow is an indicator as to whether a business is growing its cash with profits or if the profits are only on paper.

Ideally, all of the growth rates should be equal to or greater than 10 percent per year for the last 5, 3 and 1 year. Having at least these three numbers gives you a better sense of how the company is growing over a period of time. Fundamental to all of the numbers is consistency. We want all the numbers going up or at least staying the same.

I realize that this quick overview of the top 5 growth rates just gives you a smattering of what to assess. Self-made stock investment millionaire *Phil Town* pioneered the approach of using 5 fundamental growth rates to find wonderful businesses at attractive prices. He provides a detailed step-by-step process for assessing the merits of any stock in his books *Rule #1* and *Payback Time*. Can you see how these resources could make your learning that much easier?

Factor #6: Debt-to-Equity Ratio.

The debt-to-equity ratio is a simple measure of how much the company owes in relation to how much it owns. It's calculated by dividing the total liabilities by the net equity. This ratio is easy to find on most financial websites. It should be low and preferably less than 0.5.

You can also look at a company's balance sheet to determine the total amount of debt coming due over the next few years. If there is a great deal of debt, dividends from dividend-paying companies may be slashed in order to ensure paying off any bond holders first. Here's a tip. Do a quick check is to see if the long-term debt of the company can be paid off in less than 3 years with the current free cash flow or net earnings. This gives you a margin of safety in assessing the extent of debt on the company's books. Ideally, this should be zero thus enabling the business to readily respond to drastic changes in the economy. However, those businesses capable of paying off debt within a 3-year window are still good prospects to consider.

Factor #7: PEG ratio.

A helpful indicator when comparing two or more like businesses together is the PEG ratio. The PEG is the Price-to-Earnings Multiple (P/E) divided by its earnings growth rate. It is an indicator of growth at a reasonable price, or what the stock investment industry calls GARP.

The PEG is a great way to identify growth stocks that are still selling at a good price. The lower the PEG the better, since you're getting more earnings growth for every dollar invested. As a rule of thumb, healthy companies have PEG rates less than 1, whereas a PEG rate over 2 is expensive.

The PEG ratio was championed by investment guru **Peter Lynch** who generated an annualized return of 29.8 % from 1977 to 1990 from Fidelity's Magellan Fund while the S&P 500 had an average return of 15.8 %.

Factor #8: Price-to-Sales Ratio.

The price-to-sales ratio was promoted by investment guru **Ken Fisher** back in the 80's. Fisher believed that earnings can be more volatile in the traditional P/E ratio as opposed to sales which tend to rarely decline in good companies. The PSR is calculated by dividing the stock price per share by the total sales per share. This ratio can help indicate if you are paying too much for the company's stock based on its sales. This is a useful indicator when assessing retailers.

The general rule of thumb is that the lower the PSR the better. Cyclical retailers with a PSR between 0.4 and 0.8 are good investment candidates. A cyclical stock is one that does better when the economy is doing well and people have more discretionary money to spend. Noncyclical stocks with a PSR between 0.75 and 1.5 also offer good value for investors.

Factor #9: Relative Strength Index.

The RSI measures the velocity and magnitude of directional price movements in a stock. It's most typically used on a 14-day timeframe. The indicator is measured on a scale from 0 to 100, with high and low levels marked at 80 and 20, respectively.

I've included this one technical indicator of stock momentum into the mix for screening potential candidates. The reason becomes apparent based on **James O'Shaughnessy** comment in his book **What Works on Wall Street** that *"we find that relative strength is among the only pure growth factors that actually beats the market consistently, by a wide margin."*

O'Shaughnessy says to *"buy stocks with the best relative strength, but understand that their volatility will continually test your emotional endurance."* Start your initial screening by looking for stocks that have an RSI above 50 and below 80 on a 100-point scale.

Please keep in mind that the cannabis industry is a relatively new one in terms of having a long track record in the stock market. This means that many up-and-coming businesses do not have five years of financial data to base your "ideal" investment decisions on. In this case, look for potential growth trends using the selection criteria mentioned. Companies entering into joint venture projects that'll increase overall market share are good bets.

So far, so good? Moving along to what specific steps to take for your assessment process.

An overview of the stock assessment process:

Now that we have an idea as to some of the specific indicators that we can use for assessing the money-making potential of any business, it might be the time to step back and provide a quick overview of how that process will unfold.

There are three key steps to follow when picking potential stocks for your investment portfolio. Your primary objective is to analyze several businesses and determine which ones have the greatest upside potential for growth. In essence, before you commit any of your hard-earned cash to any stock purchase, you'll be doing an in-depth best-of-breed analysis of several businesses. This analysis considers the following three steps:

Step #1: Compare the fundamentals of the business over preferably a 5-year period of time. Fundamentals refer to the rate of growth of sales, income, and equity in comparison to the on-going expenses and liabilities. We've just covered nine of the most popular indicators used by many professional investors to help them select fundamentally sound stocks. Ideally, you're looking for businesses with a long track record of consistently growing owner/ shareholder equity year to year.

Step #2: Determine the type and extent of the competitive advantage or economic moat that the business has created that sets it apart from its competition. We'll explore seven types of economic moats in a moment.

Step #3: Assess the management's focus and compensation. You're looking for CEO's that are passionate about their work and the importance they place on creating real long-term sustainable value for their shareholders. Look for management teams that are fairly compensated for their efforts as opposed to the few who rip off unsuspecting shareholders with outrageous bonuses.

Since we've already explored the key fundamentals that you should consider when finding and sizing up potential candidates, we'll delve into how 7 different types of economic moats help you make money in the markets. Sound like a plan, Sam?

Seven types of economic moats to help you make money:

There are many factors you should consider when choosing those top-notch businesses that have great growth potential and are capable of generating substantial profits for you over the years. So, how important is it that a company has a well-established economic moat? The short answer: crucial.

An economic moat refers to the notion that the business has some durable competitive advantage, not unlike a moat that protects a castle from attack. The wider the moat the easier it is to fend off attackers. Finding a business with a wide moat is key to finding a successful business to own; the wider the moat, the more predictable its future 5 to 10 years down the road. Having a competitive edge, allows for a company to have a degree of predictability.

As an investor, you're looking for not only sustainable growth rates but also consistent growth in cash flow, equity and sales over a 3 to 5-year period of time. With increasing cash flow, profitability for both the business and you the shareholder arises. With increasing cash flow, a best-of-breed business can whether the ups and downs of the economic business cycle paying off debt when needed or investing capital for expanding into new markets. Wide moat companies are also protected from inflation since their "monopolistic position" enables them to raise prices at will.

Here are seven types of economic moats to look for in a potential business:

Moat #1: Brand – a product or service you're willing to pay more for because you know and trust it. Companies like Disney and Nike have good brand moats.

Moat #2: Secret - a patent, copyright or trade secret that makes competition difficult or illegal. Examples of these companies are 3M, Pfizer and Apple.

Moat #3: Toll - having exclusive control of a market through government approval or licensing thus being able to charge a "toll" for accessing that product or service. Such businesses as PG & E, a utility company and Time Warner a media business fit the mold.

Moat #4: Switching - being too much trouble to switch to another provider due to the high monetary and time costs. Microsoft and H & R Block are two good examples.

Moat #5: Low Price - products priced so low no one can compete because they enjoy massive economies of scale due to a huge market share. Home Depot, Costco and Wal-Mart are examples of businesses that have used pricing to establish an economic advantage.

Moat #6: Network Effect - the ability to quickly dominate a network of end-users by being first in the market. eBay was the first online auction business to dominate the North American market.

Moat #7: Unique Corporate Culture - a way of doing business that would be difficult to duplicate in another business environment. Southwest Airlines benefited from this type of economic moat in the early years.

You need not find a company with multiple moats to consider it to be a potential investment candidate. It should have one moat that seems hardest to cross and one that is sustainable long-term. And how do you identify an economic moat? The establishment of a viable economic moat shows up in the fundamentals. Companies with consistently high growth rates of over 10% per year in return on invested capital, sales, equity and free cash over many years are the ideal candidates.

Is management on your side?

Step 3 of your assessment process looks at who is running the company. As obvious as it may be, we want management to be on the side of the shareholder. However, this is not always the case. We've seen countless cases of incidents where the CEO did not have the shareholder's best interest at heart. Situations where the CEO is being paid hundreds of millions of dollars to run the company into the ground. Here are the top four qualities that you want to see in great CEO's:

1. They are service-oriented as opposed to ego-oriented. Their focus is on serving the owners, the employees, the suppliers, and the customers.
2. They are passionate about their work and the business they are managing.
3. They never risk their honor to make a quick buck or ruin their reputation for power or prestige.
4. They are driven to change the world for the better. They have big goals that inspire and motivate the organization.

How do you go about finding this information? Here are five ways to check out management without hiring a private eye:

1. Google the CEO's name and read a few news articles in trade and business magazines and newspapers, such as Forbes, Fortune, Barron's, Success, the New York Times and the Wall Street Journal. What reputation does the CEO have in the business community?

2. Check out the competition's websites and blogs for information about the manager and the company. What are they saying about their competition and the challenges in the market?
3. Read the CEO's letter to shareholders and compare the growth rate numbers to what is being said. What is the tone of the letter? Look for CEO's who take responsibility for a bad year, as evidenced in the numbers, admits his or her mistakes and tells shareholders what he or she intends to do. These CEO's have integrity.
4. To better understand a specific business, check out either the CEO's quarterly conference call held with analysts and recorded on the company's website or posted as a transcript of the call. A couple of hours of reading or listening every 3 months will teach you a whole lot about the CEO.
5. Look at the Insider trading activity on MSN Money or Yahoo Finance. If company executives are unloading more than 30 percent of their stock all at once, this is not a good sign. As well, look for CEO's that are getting overpaid through stock options or outrageous perks in addition to their salary. Most free websites post this basic data.

Ask yourself, does the business have great Management? You must be confident that the people running the business are doing so as if they intend on being there for decades and not out to rip you off in the short term. Does that make sense?

Once you have explored a business's fundamentals, competitive advantage and management team you can use the same approach with that business's key competitors to determine who is the best-of-breed in that industry. By identifying and investing initially in only these best-of-breed companies, especially when they come on sale at attractive prices, you increase the likelihood that you'll build a successful investment portfolio.

All of this information can be recorded either in a notebook or in an Excel Spreadsheet. Although taking a little more time to set up, a spreadsheet affords the greatest future ease of use for both the calculations and updating information. This process has served me well in assessing potential candidates. It has helped me streamline the information flow so that I am more efficient, saving me time in the process.

A simple way to calculate growth rates:

Are you wondering how you can determine or calculate the key growth rates that we discussed earlier?

Sometimes a little mental math is all that you need to perform in order to get an approximate value for a particular growth rate.

Many of you have heard of the rule of 72, which states that by dividing 72 by the number of years it takes to double your money, you end up with an approximation of the growth rate.

For example, let's say you're looking at a potential candidate with an initial Book Value per Share (BVPS) of 8 in 2007 and a final BVPS of 32 in 2017.

Step #1: See how many times the initial BVPS value in 2007 doubles in 10 years to reach or slightly surpass the final BVPS value in 2017. In other words, if the starting BVPS is 8 and the final BVPS is 32, how many times can you double 8 before reaching or slightly surpassing 32?
A BVPS of 8 doubles twice: once from 8 to 16 and then from 16 to 32. Therefore, one double takes 5 years.

Step #2: Using the "Rule of 72", divide the number of years it takes to double once into 72. That is divide 72 by 5 which is approximately 14 ½. This is your percentage rate of growth.
You now have a good estimate of the annual growth rate over 10 years.

Whichever method you decide to employ when calculating growth rates, your primary goal as an investor should be to simplify the whole process. Choose the method that best suits your needs with this in mind.

Chapter 12: Which Investment Strategies Are Right for Me?

Let's explore a handful of strategies that work well with an accelerated cash flow system. Are you fired up and ready to go? Do you know what I'm thinking? No! Neither do I; frightening isn't it?

The most important factor about strategies:

Before we take a look at the handful of time-tested strategies outlined in this book, let's take a quick look at the obvious challenge many retail investors are faced with - that of picking which strategy to use.

There are an overwhelming number of popular investment strategies being used in the stock market today. Many experts tout that they have the perfect strategy that is the be-all and end-all to solving your investment woes. Many well-known investment authors who have been successful investing in the stock market often have a strong bias towards a particular strategy that better sells their services or investment product lines.

It's challenging to get an unbiased opinion about any particular investment strategy. Who can you really trust when many of them have a hidden agenda? The American Association of Individual Investors currently tracks over 60 investment strategies on their website. It's no wonder that most do-it-yourself retail investors are at a loss as to which approach to take.

The most important aspect about making money in the markets is to <u>stick to a proven strategy over time</u>. It becomes more of a factor the longer you work your specific strategy through good times and bad. Avoid adopting the attitude that if Plan A fails, you've got 25 more letters to choose from. The handful of strategies selected for accelerating your cash flow avoids this. They create opportunities to generate a significant stream of cash flow as well as increase the velocity of your money from one opportunity to a better one.

How to create a diverse stock portfolio:

Diversification means different things to different investors. Many mutual fund advisers tout that diversification is best achieved by buying an index or basket of 100 or more stocks through some type of fund. Others in the expert arena, such as **Jim Cramer** or **Phil Town** suggest holding a handful of stocks that have been personally selected.

So, how do you create a diverse portfolio of investments that provides both upside potential and downside protection of your wealth? For the avid stock investor, here are seven key factors to integrate into your investment portfolio in order to create an appropriate level of diversification:

Factor #1: Diversification Across Asset Classes.

As a lifelong investor, your ideal investment portfolio should contain not only stocks, but also investments from other asset classes.

By investing in other asset classes such as real estate rental property, commodities like oil and gold, systematized businesses that run on their own, or fixed-income investments like bonds, you spread out your risk across various investment markets. When one market is trending lower another unrelated one may be heading higher.

Investing in various asset classes creates a better balance in preserving your overall capital and should be one of your long-term investment objectives. Most self-made millionaires use a multi-faceted approach to wealth creation and so should you.

Although we're focusing on building wealth using the stock market as a vehicle, at some point in the future you may wish to explore other investment vehicles. Makes sense, right?

Factor #2: Diversification Within the Stock Market.

When you invest in the stock market, your portfolio may benefit from being invested in various groups of stocks that are classified by size or characteristics. For example, a core amount of your investment capital will be initially invested in dividend-paying large cap stocks, with a certain percentage of your capital being spread across the small or mid cap stock universe. Each group has its own unique characteristics that benefit from certain market or economic conditions. By the way, the expression "large cap" refers to large capitalization, which is another way of saying a large business.

At times, you may find that your investments in the small-cap universe will prove to be winners in a booming economy. Most cannabis-related businesses currently fit into this category with huge profit potential in the coming years.

At other times your dividend-paying stocks may out-perform the small or mid-cap stock universes. By diversifying your capital within the stock market, you can benefit from the changing tides that occur every 4 to 6 years.

Factor #3: Diversification Across the 11 Economic Sectors.

A popular way of grouping companies traded in the stock market has been to place them into 11 economic sectors based on the nature or purpose of the business. Examples of these economic sectors are the technology sector, consumer staples, energy, utilities and health care.

By allocating no more than 20% of your investment capital to any one of the 11 economic sectors provides you with better balance. As one economic sector goes out of favor with Mr. Market, another will quickly take its place. Spreading out your capital improves your odds of overall portfolio growth.

It stands to reason that once you have a number of good investment candidates you should be aware of how you allocate your capital across the 11 sectors.

Factor #4: Diversification Across the Globe.

God created the world, everything else is made in China. Although the U.S. has the most vibrant stock markets in the world, you should actively seek out companies that have a global exposure. This can be done with U.S. based companies that export more than 30% of their goods or services overseas or through ADR's, which are foreign companies that trade on U.S. exchanges.

Look for the tag ADR, which stands for American Depository Receipt, after the name of a company you're researching. Consider exposing yourself to Canadian companies in the cannabis industry. Canada has a commodity-based economy and one of the strongest financial systems in the world.

Also take a look at the BRICS countries, Brazil, Russia, India, China and South Africa, whose growing middle class are buying more and more local products and services, not to mention those of the international players.

To start with, focus your attention on U.S. and Canadian companies with international exposure, as well as those foreign businesses listed as ADRs on the U.S. stock exchanges.

Factor #5: Diversification Across Time.

By investing on a regular basis, you're able to tap into opportunities as they present themselves. Having cash on hand to take advantage of miss pricings in the market allows you to buy into positions with a certain margin of safety.

Recall that it is the velocity of your money through the stock market from one investment to a better one that accelerates your wealth-building potential. The old adage of buy, hold and forget - no longer works in today's markets. You may be better served by moving your "dead money" into growth opportunities on a regular basis. Following me so far?

Factor #6: Diversification Across Investment Accounts.

Not all investment accounts are created equal. A few allow you to grow your investments tax-free, others defer the tax you pay, and some offer better investment choices.

You should try to diversify your holdings across 3 general types of accounts because of the advantages and limitations of each.

Many employed investors are familiar with the 401(k) [RRSP in Canada] which creates a tax deduction up front in return for taxable income once money is withdrawn at retirement. When employers are matching your contributions, it makes sense to take advantage of the match up to the allowable maximum set up by your employer.

The Roth IRA [TFSA in Canada] is a tax-free account in which investment capital that has already been taxed can grow and compound over time to be used tax free at a future date. "Self-directed" IRA [TFSA] accounts have many more investment choices beyond just a small selection of mutual funds, ETF's or bonds typically offered in 401(k) accounts.

Finally, an individual margin account allows you the greatest investment choice flexibility from stocks to options to commodities plays. This type of account gives you greater control over making money whether the market is heading up or everyone else is panicking in a sell-off. For example, since my TFSA account is maxed out for lifetime contributions, any future investment capital is directed into my margin account.

Factor #7: Diversification Across Investment Strategies.

It is well-documented that some investment strategies work better under certain economic conditions than others. Consistently using a few time-tested solid performers will help to boost your overall returns, which brings us to looking at some specific simple strategies for covered call writing.

As you can surmise, by taking into consideration these various diversification factors, you'll be in a more solid position to protect your downside while generating more consistent returns in the future.

Three effective covered call strategies:

Now it's time to take a look at how we can integrate covered call strategies into our overall cash flow plan. Unlike you, most stock investors are limited to making money only when the stock goes up in price.

Whether you're investing for the long-haul or trading stocks every few months as opportunities present themselves, the average investor can only realistically expect a historical market return of around 10% or slightly higher should they be adept at moving into and out of the market.

In real estate, an investor can buy a piece of property in the hopes that the property will increase in price over time. The concept is no different from the stock investor buying a particular stock in the hopes that it too will go up in price. The real estate investor can create a monthly cash flow by renting out his investment. In exchange for a roof over one's head, the real estate investor is paid a monthly rent.

The stock investor can also rent out his stock in the form of covered call options. However, there's no roof over one's head in this situation. The stock investor can receive cash up front in exchange for the right to buy the stock from you should it reach an agreed upon price.

When you become a covered call writer, someone who rents out their stock in exchange for a monthly or bi-monthly rental premium, your ability to generate additional profits under varying market conditions increases. You can make money when the stock goes up to your agreed upon rental price or what is known as the strike price. This occurs most often in an upward trending or bullish market. You'll often capture both the rental premium and any stock price appreciation between your initial price and the strike price.

You can make money when the stock goes nowhere by capturing the rental premium. This occurs when the markets or the stock are neutral or flat over a period of time.

You can also protect your money better should the stock experience a slight drop in price over the course of a month or so. When a stock or the market is bearish and trending lower, covered calls offer some downside protection of your stock price. This is accomplished by having your rental premium lowering your initial cost basis for the stock, thus providing a slight cushion against loss of capital.

As you can see, the selling of covered calls, increases your ability to generate additional cash flow from your investments. Under normal market conditions, a covered call writer can expect a monthly return in the range of 2 to 4% in additional to any stock price appreciation. Given that you could realistically expect to sell monthly calls almost every month that equates to annual potential returns in excess of 20 to 30%. Wouldn't you like to get your hands on that little puppy?

The challenge now becomes in learning a few strategies that allow you to consistently capture those gains. When you just buy and sell stocks, the time commitment is usually minimal. You may spend a lot of time initially picking your stocks, but once you purchase those shares there is usually a minimal amount of ongoing weekly monitoring.

On the other hand, selling covered calls on your stock holdings requires another layer of monitoring above and beyond the time required for stock selection. You'll need to watch your positions on a daily basis. However, you'll only be spending a few minutes on each position to monitor the stock price in relation to the option price.

You'll also need to spend a little bit of time planning and preparing your exit and entry strategies on a monthly basis. This small investment in time each week and at the end of each month is well worth the massive increase in cash flow you could experience by being actively engaged in making money in the markets.

The purpose of the following section is to do just that - provide you with four simple covered call strategies that you can use to accelerate your cash flow from stock investing. But, before we get into the nitty gritty of selling covered calls, let's take a look at a few concepts that you should be familiar with in order to better understand how you can use each of these strategies.

Options basics:

When you sell any option contract, besides selecting the specific stock, there will be four conditions that you will need to fill in before your order is fulfilled. These four requirements are:

Condition #1: The strike price.

This is the price that you agree to sell your stock at should the price of the stock reach this specific price at any time before the contract expires. In theory, your shares of stock could be sold at any time the stock price is at or higher than your agreed upon strike price. However, the majority of the time, the sale of your shares, what is called assignment or exercising your shares, happens on the last day of the contract known as expiration Friday. Expiration Friday is always the 3rd Friday of the expiration month.

The strike price that you select can be above, at or below the current price of the stock. When the strike price is above the current price, it is known as an out-of-the-money call or OTM. When the strike price is at the current price, it is known as an at-the-money call or ATM. When the strike price is below the current price, it is known as an in-of-the-money call or ITM.

Condition #2: The contract expiration date.

Each option contract has a limited life expectancy that is stipulated as the contract expiration date. For a seller of options contracts (that's you) this is an advantage especially when the contract period is short as in a 1-month time frame. The most successful and consistent covered call writers like to work with monthly contracts.

As time passes there is a natural erosion of the value of an options contract, which eventually falls to zero at the end of the trading day on expiration Friday.

Condition #3: The number of contracts.

Option contracts are sold in whole number lots, where each contract controls 100 shares of stock. No fractional units or shares of stock are allowed. For example, if you have 455 shares of Cannabis Wheaton stock, the maximum number of covered call contracts that you can sell is 4. You're unable to write a contract for the remaining 55 shares. This is why I make a strong case for trying to purchase stock in round lots of 100 shares so that you can optimize your option positions.

Condition #4: The premium price.

The total premium that you receive as a call seller is composed of two parts - value that is associated with time and intrinsic value.

To better illustrate this concept, let's take a look at a few simplified call-selling scenarios.

If you were to sell an at-the-money (ATM) call option contract at the beginning of the month for $2 with a strike price of $45 when the current stock price is hovering around $45, your premium paid would be made up of $2 of time value. This time value is based on the appreciation potential of the option. This appreciation potential takes into consideration both the time left until contract expiration and the volatility of the stock as it trades.

Here's a 2nd scenario. Should you have settled for a strike price of $46, which is above the current stock price, in other words we sold an out-of-the-money (OTM) call for $1; it would be made up only of time value, nothing else. Your total premium paid to you would be made up of only the potential for option appreciation by a specified date. And this premium would get smaller the further out-of-the-money you sell your option contract for.

Now let's assume in our 3rd scenario that you sell an in-the-money (ITM) call with a strike of $43 when the stock price is $45, and you receive a premium of $4. Notice that the option contract is now worth $2 more, having increased in value from $2 to $4, when we looked at our initial ATM call. This second part that makes up the total premium is attributed to intrinsic value. Intrinsic value just tells you if the option has any true or real value. It's related to how much a particular option is in-the-money giving us some actual tangible value. In this case, the call option is now $2 in-the-money.

Another way of looking at intrinsic value is that the further in-the-money the option is the greater it's intrinsic value. This value is approximately equal to the number of dollars that the stock price is in-the-money.

Yes, I realize that this is an over-simplification of the premium calculation process. My intent is to illustrate the relationship between time and intrinsic value. In the real world, the time value component would probably have adjusted downwards slightly due to the effects of time erosion on the option contract.

To recap, the four basic parameters that you will need to initially input after selecting your specific stock when you sell a covered call contract are:

1. Strike price.
2. Expiration date.
3. Number of contracts.
4. Premium price.

When you're in your online discount brokerage account, you're best served by placing a "limit" order that is good for the day for your option order rather than sending the order in as a "market" order. By placing a limit price for your orders, you have greater control over the price you could end up initially selling your contracts at and also the price you're willing to buy them back at, if necessary, as part of your exit strategy. We'll look at this and other timing strategies in greater detail for entering and exiting the market in the following section.

Now that we have an idea as to which parameters we need to enter for each call option position that we undertake, let's take a look at three simple call selling strategies to place in your investment arsenal. Please keep in mind that these strategies are not carved in stone. As with any strategy, they are to be used as a guideline in helping you make the best investment choices that'll accelerate your cash flow and provide some protection of your capital.

To see how each of these strategies unfolds with real life examples, check out *Alan Ellman's* short video tutorials on You Tube at his Blue Collar Investor channel. I find that a visual presentation to be the most effective learning tool. Use the following information in this book to get a feel for the strategies and the pros and cons of using each one.

Since markets trend upwards over time, let's take an initial look at how you can tap into stocks that are showing some price appreciation.

Option strategy #1: Growth generation in up-trending markets.

A growth strategy for call options is one that allows for both gains to be made in the stock price appreciation, as well as premium received from selling your calls. It requires that you sell an out-of-the-money call (OTM).

Growth Generation Strategy Advantages.

There are three major advantages of using the growth generation strategy, namely:

1. You profit from both the option premium received and the upside appreciation of the stock.
2. You have less of a chance of your stock being assigned and called away (i.e. cashed out) at the end of the option cycle since the stock price has further to rise than an at-the-money call option strategy.
3. Time decay works in your favor since there is no intrinsic value, only time value. As time lapses, the option premium approaches zero, accelerating even faster just days prior to expiration Friday.

Growth Generation Strategy Disadvantages.

The top three disadvantages are that:

1. You have the least amount of downside protection should the stock decline in value, since there is no intrinsic value had you bought an in-the-money call.
2. You'll probably receive an initial premium that is low. The further away the strike price is from the current stock price the lower the premiums. An at-the-money call yields you the highest "initial" premiums.
3. You'll probably pay more to close your position should the stock price drop. This is due to the relationship between stock price and option price.

Option strategy #2: Income generation in neutral markets.

An income strategy for call options is one that attempts to capture high premiums from your call selling. You'll usually be selling at-the-money calls (ATM).

Income Generation Strategy Advantages.

There are two major advantages of using the income generation strategy, namely:
1. It provides the highest initial option return resulting in a pure income generation play.
2. It takes advantage of maximizing immediate cash flow into your brokerage account.

Income Generation Strategy Disadvantages.

The top three disadvantages are that:
1. You have no upside potential for stock price appreciation.
2. There is also no downside protection as with an in-the-money call position.
3. You have a high probability of stock being called away (sold).

Option strategy #3: Protection strategy in down-trending markets.

A protection strategy for call options is one that attempts to capture premiums from your call selling as well as cushion your cash basis in your stock should the stock price decline slightly over the course of the month. This involves selling in-the-money calls (ITM).

Protection Strategy Advantages

There are three major advantages of using the protection strategy, namely:
1. You receive immediate option profit from the sale of the call.
2. The position creates downside protection for your stock price.
3. This is a lower risk strategy compared to the other call option strategies.

Protection Strategy Disadvantages

The top three disadvantages are that:
1. You have no upside potential.
2. There are lost opportunity costs since you do not participate in any potential for share appreciation.
3. You have a high probability of the stock being called away on or before expiration Friday.

Now that you have a brief idea as to how you could use covered calls for three specific investment situations, it's time to look at some totally trippin tips.

Top 15 covered call strategy tips:

To wrap up this section on selling calls, here are my top 15 strategy tips for writing covered calls on stock that you own. Even though, you've seen some of these key concepts before, they're worth repeating and re-stating with a slightly different perspective.

Tip #1: Learn before you earn.

Don't invest in anything you do not understand. No matter what your investment strategy, take the time to learn the basics so that you can make appropriate investment decisions. I encourage you to tap into the wealth of knowledge being shared by some of the educators mentioned in this book. Check out your Appendix for resources to explore down the road.

Tip #2: Keep your options investment system simple.

Keep your technical analysis as simple and easy as possible. I only use a handful of technical indicators to guide my decision-making. Also, avoid using time intensive systems. If you are having to personally track and update a myriad of multiple variables on a daily basis, start looking for an easier approach. Life is too short to be pre-occupied with your investments, day in and day out. Wouldn't you agree?

Tip #3: Spread out your capital.

Don't put all of your eggs in one basket. You should have no more than 20% of your investment capital in any one industry and preferably spread across the 11 economic sectors. Industries can go out of favor very quickly. You should also spread out your capital across investment strategies to optimize your portfolio for consistent profitability.

Having a rigid money-management system in place allows me to both preserve my capital and maintain a high level of confidence in my abilities. I plan to be in the options trading business for years to come; therefore, I know that there will be hundreds of profitable positions that I'll be able to participate in over time. No need to rush the journey and risk my hard-earned dollars.

Tip #4: Use an online discount broker where ever possible.

Full service brokerage fees will quickly erode your returns on your investments. If you trade options several times per month the high transaction costs of a full-service broker will also negatively impact your trading decisions by having you hold onto positions longer than you should because you don't want to incur the big fees.

Tip #5: Always pick stocks for options trading that are fundamentally sound.

Whether you use the selection criteria outlined in this guide or criteria from a reputable source, always seek the best of breed businesses within a specific industry. You can make a lot more money with options plays by choosing companies that have a proven track record for growth especially if they are market leaders.

Tip #6: Monitor your holdings on a regular basis.

This enables you to optimize your profits by using appropriate exit strategies when the time comes. You need not spend an inordinate amount of time verifying the fundamentals and looking at a technical chart of your positions. However, you do need to be positioned to take advantage of money-making opportunities as they present themselves.

Tip #7: Learn to use a variety of options strategies, not just one.

For example, don't just sell out-of-the money covered calls just because they're one of the most popular options strategies. Base your investment decisions on the direction and mood of the market, as well as what the current technicals are indicating for a particular opportunity play.

Tip #8: Watch the greed factor.

Don't sell covered calls that generate excessively high monthly returns. Your sweet spot for monthly returns should be in the range of 2 to 4%; anything higher than 5% may be a sign of higher stock volatility.

Tip #9: Avoid selling covered calls on stocks that have a quarterly earnings report during the same month.

Earnings reports can create excessive volatility whereby the stock is now trading over a much wider price range. Better to watch the stock over the month and re-evaluate its suitability after the earnings report is public.

Tip #10: Be mindful of transaction fees.

Try to sell (rent out) at least 4 or 5 contracts (1 option contract = 100 shares of stock) at a time in order to reduce the effects of commissions decreasing your net premium. The fewer the contracts being sold; the more commissions will begin to erode your premium profits.

As a general word of caution, avoid selling covered calls in rapidly rising or falling markets. These markets are rare, occurring every 4 to 6 years, so most of the time, covered call writing is an appropriate strategy.

A rapidly declining market is best handled by sidestepping out of the stock market and moving your cash into other opportunities in possibly other asset classes or by waiting patiently in a cash or cash-equivalent position for opportunities to present themselves. On the other hand, in a rapidly rising market, you may be better served through the natural appreciation of the stock price, especially if it exceeds our 2 to 4% monthly covered call expectation.

Tip #11: Always assess the business's fundamentals, technical indicators and your mental state before placing a trade.

I ensure that all of my geese are properly lined up before placing any trade. This not only builds confidence, it also creates a better edge and higher probability of coming out on top. I also never trade on a hot tip. Take the time to do your due diligence on each potential trade. It'll have a dramatic effect on your bottom line.

Tip #12: Determine both an entry point and exit point for each opportunity.

When you pre-plan your trades, you increase your probability of success. Entering a trade when you have had a chance to clearly think through possible outcomes should be your objective every time you place a trade. Getting caught up in the excitement of the market at a specific unanticipated moment could spell disaster. Thinking through rational outcomes in advance increases your chances of pulling off a winning transaction. This thinking process takes into consideration how much capital is at risk and what specific trading parameters either increase risk or mitigate it.

Tip #13: Take full responsibility for your actions.

Do not blame the weather, your neighbor's dog or Mr. Market for the outcome of a particular investment decision. Always remember that every potential investment opportunity is unique. Learn from the mistakes that you'll inevitably make, but do not dwell on the negative outcome. All investors make errors that cost them money. I know have. How else was I going to learn what works for me and doesn't?

Your goal should be to reduce the number of errors that you can control yourself over time. Re-focus your energy and time looking for the next potential opportunity. When you look at the market as being the enemy, you take yourself out of the constant flow of opportunities that present themselves. By freeing up your mind you can now focus on moving into and out of better and better opportunities.

Tip #14: Do not place a trade if you're emotionally upset, in a euphoric mood or under above average stress from your work/home environment.

When my emotional state is out of whack with my normal operating state, I tend to make silly mistakes that cost me money in the end. By tuning into my emotional state prior to each trade, I've been able to increase my ability to consistently place winning trades, while minimizing or eliminating common trading errors completely.

Tip #15: Optimize not maximize each trade.

It is okay for me to leave money on the table. I know that opportunities present themselves every month. The key is to patiently wait for those situations where you have an edge and then move back into the market taking profits when they present themselves and not feel bad if you don't maximize your profit potential.

Chapter 13: How Could I Better Time Entering & Exiting Positions?

Contrary to what many in the investment landscape are saying about timing the market, you can learn to be more adept at moving into and out of positions so that you increase the probability of coming out on top.

One of the most frustrating aspects of stock investing is trying to figure out when you should move into and out of positions. It can take you years to figure out what time periods you should avoid based on the documented historical trends. It can also take the average investor years to figure out how the movement of the big institutional players affects one's ability to profit from the entry and exit points in the market.

You will in all likelihood NOT be able to time the market tops and bottoms, thus enabling you to maximize your profits. No one has been able to consistently do this in the stock market.

However, we can take advantage of certain times of the day, week, month or year that enable us to better optimize our profits. This knowledge helps us create our "edge" thereby increasing our profitability potential in the stock market. Ready to pick up some tips?

Top ten timing tips to generating better returns:

The following are my top ten tips to better timing the market and more importantly why.

Tip #1: Avoid buying stock or call options on a Monday.

If you decide to move into a position on Monday morning, expect higher than normal price volatility throughout the day. According to former trading floor boss *Joe Terranova* in his book *Buy High Sell Higher*: *"Whether traders love or hate their personal lives, the pros that move the market often come into the office on Mondays in a bad mood. Whatever the reason, there is always a flood of emotion coursing through the market on Mondays. Markets that are trading on emotions are not where you want to be. I make a point of never trading on Mondays."*

I tend to concur with *Joe*. You as a cash flow investor are better served by waiting for the markets to play out during the course of the day on Mondays. They tend to be too emotionally charged after the weekend.

Tip #2: Try to trade on Wednesdays and Thursdays.

On the flip side of the coin is to ask yourself when would be the ideal time to try to better time my market plays? Mid-week tends to present better investment opportunities than either the beginning or end of the week. According to *Jeffrey Hirsch* in his book the *Stock Trader's Almanac* Wednesday's have produced the most gains since 1990.

Often on Fridays many big institutional players unload certain positions before the weekend, preferring not to hold potentially volatile stocks that may be affected by news over the weekend. This coupled with the notion that many traders take off early on Friday afternoon means that the smaller players become the temporary price movers. Watch to see that the price movement of the stock is in synch with the volume of shares being traded. A rising stock price yet decreasing volume is a signal that the current stock price trend is unsustainable over time.

Tip #3: Avoid trading first thing in the morning and during the lunch hour.

As to what time of the day may present better buy and sell opportunities, you may be best served by waiting at least an hour or so after the opening bell before getting into the market. I have made this mistake a couple of times, only to realize later in the morning that I overpaid for my positions. Another time of the day that may be problematic is midday during the lunch hour when many professional traders take their lunch. With fewer traders, market volume tends to lag.

A little patience as to seeing how the day may be unfolding may save you a few bucks in the end. By waiting until the end of the day when volume is typically the heaviest, you may be in a better position to assess your timing opportunity. Remember that above average volume with rising stock prices is a signal that investors are confident in a particular stock or the market as a whole.

Tip #4: Avoid trading at the end or beginning of a quarter.

Be very attentive as to stocks that you may be holding which have been lack luster over the past quarter. Many institutional players unload poor performers in an attempt to re-balance their overall portfolio. Keep in mind that the mutual fund industry is very competitive and that many fund managers take a short-term approach to investing in order to hang onto their client's money.

By being vigilant at the end of each quarter you can better assess the impact of buying or selling particular holdings based on what you feel the big boys may be doing. Sometimes you can get a feel for the tone of the market as a whole by watching how money is flowing into the stock market as opposed to bond market or commodities such as gold and oil.

Tip #5: Avoid trading when company earnings are announced.

The time period just leading up to and soon after an earnings report release can see volatile stock price movement. Earnings reports can signal shifts in momentum. This is especially important when you'll be selling covered calls on the stock during the same month that earnings are going to be announced.

It may be more prudent to wait out the period around the earnings report release to see how Mr. Market will handle the information rather than commit yourself to a call position. You can always take up a position once you're assured that the news will not have a negative effect on your positions.

Tip #6: Be wary of the first 2 to 3 weeks of January.

Many companies have year-end earnings announcements in January, which can translate to increased stock price volatility.

The large institutional players typically have major capital allocation flows in and out of stocks during this period of time. This is especially so with the commodity-based funds. If you've identified a commodity-based stock that you would like to invest in, you may be better served waiting on the sidelines until the big boys have finished their dance with increased price volatility.

I'm guilty of making this mistake. Instead of being more patient with purchasing a particular stock, I ended up initially paying more for the investment as the stock dropped in price mid-January. I had to wait on the sidelines for a short period of time until April for the stock to appreciate up to a level that I felt comfortable selling option contracts at.

As you know, the name of the game is increasing the velocity of your money. Unfortunately, my money was parked in a position whereby I was unable to generate a monthly cash flow. Bad boy, R.J.. You should to be taken out behind the wood shed for a licking.

Tip #7: Schedule any important moves after mid-April.

The stock market tends to be more prone to weakness after the mid-month tax deadline in the United States. This may be the result of individual investor money moving out of the markets in order to pay for tax obligations owing and the rebalancing of portfolios in order take advantage of certain capital losses.

For your own personal finances, you may wish to hold off any major moves that could have an impact on your current tax liabilities owing. It may be prudent to check with a financial planner or accountant prior to making any such big moves.

Tip #8: Be cautious investing in early October.

The beginning of October has often been weak for the stock market. There tends to be fewer growth plays during this particular time period. The markets typically ramp up for the Christmas season come late October or early November.

You may wish to keep closer tabs on the market by following the fall trend of the S&P 500 Index and those specific sectors you're currently interested in. More on that in a moment.

Tip #9: Be aware of sector rotations.

Some sectors and industries show strength at certain times of the year. Large institutional players tend to support certain sectors at specific times of the year.

For example, the technology sector and consumer discretionary are usually stronger in the fall and weaker in spring. This aligns well with the expected increase in consumer spending that occurs from October to January every year.

Another example is that of the oil refiners who tend to do well in the first and fourth quarters of the year as demand for heating oil increases over the winter months.

Tip #10: Avoid the investo-tainment hype.

This is a tough tip to follow. It is counter-intuitive to not jump on the investing bandwagon when everyone else is singing praise for a specific stock or group of stocks. While screening for great potential stock candidates your judgment can be clouded and influenced by what you see and hear in the media.

However, you're better served by following a specific decision-making process. That process should consider analyzing a handful of key fundamentals of the business as well as the technical charts and indicators that show you when you should enter the market.

By stepping back and taking the time to process the basic data that really matters in executing your specific investment strategy, you'll save yourself a lot of grief and heartache knowing that you haven't been duped by the investo-tainment hype.

One question that has served me well when I see excessive posturing for a particular stock in the media is: What are other investors thinking about regarding this recent news and how are they going to react to the recent media attention? By thinking socially, I'm in a better position to build my edge and increase the probability of making money from the opportunity.

How to place your option sell order:

After you have selected the appropriate option strategy that you would like to layer on top of your stock position, you'll need to log into your brokerage account to check out the option premiums available. The list of option strike prices and corresponding premiums is known as the option chain.

Depending on the strategy that you have selected, or will be selecting based on further analysis, you should do an initial calculation of the option return of those 2 or 3 strike prices closest to the current price of the stock. This enables you to have a better perspective of the profitability potential of at least a couple of strike prices.

Look at the current bid price, the lower price, for each option strike price to get a feel for the potential premium you might receive. Ideally, we would like to sell the selected strike price at a price that is between the bid and mid-price for that option. The mid-price is the price half way between the bid and ask prices. Some websites provide this calculation for you or you can simply do the math in your head or "guestimate" the mid price.

Once you have the stock price, the strike prices and the corresponding bid prices, enter this information into an option analysis spreadsheet. A simple spreadsheet can quickly calculate the immediate return that you'll generate from the sale of your option contracts.

The return on your option is calculated by dividing the premium received by the cost basis of your stock. Should you be selling an in-the-money option for some downside protection, the intrinsic value (i.e. protection) is deducted from the option premium before calculating the return. For example, if the stock option is $1 and the stock price is $50, your return on option (ROO) is: $1/($50-$1) = 2.0%.

As previously mentioned, the spreadsheet developed by **Owen Sargent** and used extensively by **Alan Ellman** author of **Exit Strategies for Covered Calls** can be downloaded from the Blue Collar Investor website.

It's at this point that you'll need to decide which option strike price that you'll sell. Simply log into your brokerage account and select the specific option that you would like to sell, enter the number of contracts, place a "sell to open" limit order good for the day, at a price between the bid and mid prices for the option. Hit the place order button. And check your order status in several minutes.

Once executed (the contracts are sold), record the actual premium that you received in either your trading diary or in a spreadsheet that will track your positions. And should your sell order not be filled as quickly as you would like, go into your brokerage account and "modify" your limit order so that it more closely mirrors the most recent bid price.

Exit strategies: Ten times to sell your stock.

There are many compelling reasons as to why you "could' sell one of your holdings. However, there are few reasons that justify why you really "should" cash out of your position. So, when is an "appropriate" time to sell a stock?

Consider these top 10 reasons why you might close out a position:
Reason #1: Exceptional Stock Growth.

Consider cashing out when your stock has done well and appreciated above your target price, for example having realized a 50% growth in the appreciation of the stock price. It may be appropriate to take some money off of the table and look for the next winning investment.

Reason #2: Poor Business.

If the company fundamentals have changed for the worse and the stock is tanking, you're better off quickly cutting your losses and repositioning your capital. Remember we don't want dead money sitting around. Get out and get into something that has a higher probability of generating better returns.

Reason #3: Poor Performance.

Similar to #2, if you find that the stock is not keeping up with the rest of the market over time and a better opportunity presents itself, jump at it.

Reason #4: Dividend Cuts.

Consider selling any dividend-paying stock if the dividend is cut or eliminated, which may be a red flag that the company will generate less income. Do so only if the general market is not experiencing a major correction.

Reason #5: Can't Sleep.

When you've reached your risk tolerance level and your holding is keeping you up at night, it may be time to liquidate your position and re-evaluate your investment portfolio. I did this with an options play that I was uncomfortable with from the get-go. Despite taking a loss, I was able to sleep better, refocus my energy and find a better opportunity that I was very happy to be in.

Reason #6: Reached Your Goal.

It would be appropriate to move your capital when you've achieved a specific financial goal in the markets and would like to buy a house, fund a college education or build a business.

Reason #7: Opportunity Knocks.

At times, you may need the cash for another investment opportunity such as rental real estate, a systematized business or an angel capital investment. Remember that your focus is on accelerating the velocity of your money from one great opportunity to a better one. Keep an open mind to any and all future possibilities that get you closer to realizing your dreams that much faster.

Reason #8: Retirement.

Should you be in the enviable position to retire, you may wish to shift some of your capital into other assets during retirement or use some of your capital to periodically fund part of your retirement.

Reason #9: Portfolio Out of Whack.

If your stock investment portfolio gets out of balance and you find that you're too heavily weighted in one industry or sector, it may be prudent to sell your position. Reducing your overall portfolio risk should always be in the back of your mind. Preserving your hard-earned capital is paramount.

Reason #10: Unexpected Expense.

As a last resort. you may be faced with an unexpected medical bill or emergency that requires you to liquidate your stock holding. Not an ideal situation to be faced with, but nevertheless an appropriate one should it arise.

There you have it a list of the top 10 times that you may want to consider when selling one of your positions. Your primary objective should be to generate cash flow from better and better investment opportunities. Now that you have an idea as to possible scenarios for selling a particular stock holding, let's take a look at various exit strategies for your covered call positions.

Exit strategies: Buying to close a covered call position.

Let's start by taking a look at how you close out an opening position. When you sell a covered call on stock that you own, you enter a "sell to open" transaction on your trading platform.

When you are ready to buy back your position, preferably at a lower price than what you sold the calls for, you enter a "buy to close" order with your online broker. Typically, you will select a limit order that is at the "ask price" or between the ask and the mid-price for that particular option. Recall that the ask price is the higher price between the bid and ask prices posted on the brokerage site. The entire process is the opposite of what you would expect when we sold our options contracts at the lower bid price.

When to Buy-to-Close a Call Position:

Here are four guidelines to follow as to when you could place a "buy to close" order:

Guideline #1: Stock is in danger anytime.

Place a "buy to close" order anytime the business shows major weakness in the fundamentals and the stock price could drop dramatically as a result. You want to preserve as much of your hard-earned capital as possible. Therefore, buy back your calls at any price, sell the stock and immediately move the cash into another position that is more deserving from your watch list of potential plays.

Guideline #2: Capture an 80% gain within the first couple of weeks.

If the current option premium drops below 20 percent of the initial premium that you received, buy back the contracts. This allows you the opportunity to capture the gains and be in a position to take advantage of another options play opportunity. This opportunity could occur in the same stock as it jumps back in price or it could be with another stock. Remember that the name of the game is cash flow and being able to accelerate your money through the stock market by taking advantage of better and better opportunities.

I like to set a stop loss order for my option contracts at 20% of the initial value that I sold the contracts for. I keep this standing order open until I choose to cancel or modify it. This is the one time that I consistently use stop loss orders - on my option contracts - but not on my stock holdings.

Guideline #3: Capture a 90% gain in week 3.

Should the current option premium drop below 10 percent of the original premium paid, close out your position and take your money off of the table. If your contract cycle happens to be 5 weeks long, consider buying back your option position in weeks 3 or 4. With less time left for another option play before contract expiration you should try to capture a little more in profit to compensate for the lack of time remaining. A reasonable level is to increase your expectation from 80 to 90 percent.

At the beginning of week 3, I like to reset (modify) my option stop-loss orders to reflect the new 10 percent limit. I usually keep the stop loss order "good until the close" GTC on expiration Friday.

Guideline #4: Change in stock or market tone in week 4.

There may be times when circumstances dictate that the prudent course of action is to close out your option position during the last week of the option cycle rather than do nothing and wait. You may feel that it's necessary to close out your position if the market tone changes quickly.

Should the stock show signs of weakness in its fundamentals and technicals, you might be better off exiting your position right away rather than waiting until expiration Friday. You'll want to try and convert potentially dead money into cash as soon as possible.

On the flip side, the stock may have appreciated in price above your previously sold strike price and you would like to hang onto it rather than have it called away by expiration Friday. By closing your position and simultaneously selling the next month's strike generally at or above the current stock price you can maintain control over your position.

Rolling is a common option exit strategy whereby you close out your current position and immediately sell another position. This is typically done part way through the current month's option contract with the sale of option contracts set up for the next month.

If you're interested in learning the ins and outs of covered call writing, I would suggest investing in resources that walk you through the whole process in greater detail. Check out the suggested resources at the back of this book for ideas.

Basic Option Timing Guideline:

The following is a simple guideline that I use for my investment decisions that may prove useful to you. These numbers are not carved in stone; however, they do provide you with a starting point from which to base your decisions as to which strategy may be the most appropriate. Play with the numbers as you see fit depending on your comfort level for risk, your current skill set and the time that you realistically have available for your investing.

My simple approach looks at what the monthly appreciation is for the S&P 500. I like to use the SPY ETF for my analysis, as follows:

1. If >3% = Hold onto your stock and rub your hands together like a giddy child.
2. 1% to 3% = Sell OTM calls - focus on growth.
3. Flat ± 1% = Sell ATM calls or ITM calls - focus on income.
4. -1% to -3% = Sell ITM calls - focus on protection.
5. < -3% = Move to cash &/or Buy a dividend stock.

You've now been empowered to become a better investor. This section should provide you with a boost of additional confidence that'll help you achieve your financial dreams that much faster. Wouldn't that be awesome?

Your daily routine:

Ideally, you'll want to check on your positions twice a day. Taking 10 - 15 minutes in the morning and at the end of the day should keep you abreast of what is happening in the market and hopefully keep you out of any serious trouble.

First things first. After you've had your green drink smoothie, tall glass of water or cup of java in the morning, log into your online broker account. Ah coffee! The sweet balm by which many of us accomplish tasks. Sorry, I digress.

You could also check out how the overall markets are doing at websites such as FinViz or Yahoo Finance.

Step #1: Review the overall market sentiment and any global news that may affect your current holdings.

Step #2: Review the news for each stock that you're holding. If the news is positive, think about how you could capture any gains. And if the news is negative, consider an appropriate exit strategy. Also check each stock's technical chart to verify if there were any gaps overnight that could affect your current strategy.

Step #3: Take any appropriate action if need be.

Step #4: Towards the end of the trading day around 3:30 PM EST, review the news to see if there is anything negative that might affect your positions. If you're unable to do so right before the markets close, at least verify how your holdings are doing later that evening.

Step #5: Take a quick look at a technical chart for each stock to make sure that they're behaving according to your trading plan.
Step #6: Take any appropriate action if need be. Depending on what the situation is, you may wish to wait a day or so to see if it resolves itself.

Your quarterly review:

Ever stop to think and forget to start again? You may be wondering about how you should go about monitoring your progress in your stock portfolios. Your online discount broker may be posting the daily change in your portfolio like mine does.

For the most part, I ignore this data. I'm not too concerned about knowing the day-to-day changes that occur. What I'm more interested in is the monthly flow of cash that occurs. And since this flow moves like an ocean wave, I look at my quarterly progress.

There are two metrics I'm most interested in. The first is how much cash I've been able to generate during the quarter from my options plays. In other words, what is the return on my options (ROO). Not only do I like to know if my portfolio is generating a decent monthly return of hopefully 2 - 3%, I'm also interested in the dollar value that's associated with this return.

The second metric that I like to track is has my portfolio appreciated in value over the quarter or lost some ground?

Keep in mind that the stock market moves up and down over the course of a week or month not unlike an ocean wave. This is why checking your portfolio performance on a quarterly basis makes more sense than a daily or weekly assessment.

Recall that when you control a number of options contracts, you can still generate a positive flow of cash into your brokerage account despite having a portfolio of stocks that have lost some "book" value. It's not until you sell those shares that you actually realize a loss.

This notion is encouraging because it illustrates that you can make money in the stock market despite the market going through a short correction period. A case in point is one of my own portfolios that lost book value in early 2018, yet I was able to continue having a positive cash flow with my options contracts. Wouldn't you feel more confident if this scenario played out for your portfolio?

The choice is yours right now. You can let life happen to you. Or you can embrace the wealth of insights, advice and strategies in this book and begin building life on your terms. I hope that you choose to act today and begin increasing the velocity of your money in the stock market. If you mastered some of these skills, where would you be 5 years from now.

Ready to get started?

Review Request:

Before you go, I'd like to thank you for investing in **Everything CBD**. I know that you could have picked from dozens of books on cannabis. So, a big thank you for selecting this book and reading all the way to the end.

If you enjoyed this book or if you found that you've gained greater insights into how you could conceivably build a better lifestyle, then I'd be very grateful if you'd post a positive review on Amazon.

Your support really does matter and it really does make a difference. The feedback and encouragement will help me continue to write the kind of books that help you get results.

If you'd like to leave a review, then all you need to do is go to the customer review section on the book's Amazon page. You'll then see a big button that says: "Write a customer review" - click that and you're good to go.

Thanks again for your support. To your ongoing success.

R.J

Meet R.J.

R.J. is a fun-loving, espresso-drinking, outdoor enthusiast who has travelled extensively across North America, the Caribbean and Europe.

His love of teaching has taken him into the corporate world, universities and public-school systems across Canada. He holds bachelor's degrees in both Education and Physical Education. R.J. was instrumental in changing how language programs were being delivered in the business world in Quebec where he had a language and communication company geared towards creating tailor-made courses.

Since retiring from the teaching profession, R.J. has been developing multi-media online programs for the financial and health care arenas. He loves seeing others develop healthy lifestyle habits that have a huge impact on the quality of their lives. This fuels his personal passion for sharing his interests in fitness and using more natural approaches to managing one's health challenges.

When R.J. is not having fun learning about his passions for travel, the wine industry and the health sector, he can be found hiking, mountain biking, kayaking and cross-country skiing in the Pacific Northwest with his wife. When they're taking some down time, you'll see them enjoying the outdoors by being physically active in the company of Mother Nature, whether it be exploring extensive underground cave systems in Cancun, horseback riding in the ocean in Jamaica, or scuba diving off the coast of the Grand Caymans.

They've also been known to sip on the occasional glass of Barolo wine with good friends while preparing some of their favorite Italian dishes. Above all - they enjoy living life to the fullest and creating lasting memories. They hope that this guide will empower you to do the same.

Disclaimer

This book was produced with the goal of providing information that is as accurate and reliable as possible. Regardless, purchasing this book can be seen as consent to the fact that both the publisher and the author of this book are in no way experts on the topics discussed within and that any recommendations or suggestions that are made herein are for entertainment purposes only. Professionals should be consulted as needed prior to undertaking any of the action endorsed herein.

This declaration is deemed fair and valid by both the American Bar Association and the Committee of Publishers Association and is legally binding throughout the United States.

Furthermore, the transmission, duplication or reproduction of any of the following work including specific information will be considered an illegal act irrespective of if it is done electronically or in print. This extends to creating a secondary or tertiary copy of the work or a recorded copy and is only allowed with express written consent from the Publisher. All additional rights reserved.

The information presented is broadly considered to be a truthful and accurate account of facts and as such any inattention, use or misuse of the information in question by the reader will render any resulting actions solely under their purview. There are no scenarios in which the publisher or the original author of this work can be in any fashion deemed liable for any hardship or damages that may befall them after undertaking information described herein.

Additionally, the information in this book is intended only for informational purposes and should thus be thought of as universal. As befitting its nature, it is presented without assurance regarding its prolonged validity or interim quality. Trademarks that are mentioned are done without written consent and can in no way be considered an endorsement from the trademark holder.

Appendix

Buying and Using Cannabis Related Products:

Most of these product links are for items listed on the world's largest online retailer Amazon. Use them to help you learn more about specific product or equipment options available to you. I would encourage you to shop local whenever possible should what you're looking for be competitively priced.

1. Digital Scale: https://www.amazon.com/dp/B00ME8VI34
2. Cannabis Herb Grinder: https://www.amazon.com/dp/B01BYHIENC
3. Glass Smoking Pipe: https://www.amazon.com/dp/B07GVNP42H
4. Pax 3 Vaporizer: https://www.paxvapor.com/pax-3/
5. Firefly 2: https://www.thefirefly.com/firefly-portable-vaporizer.html/
6. Herb-E Vape Pen: https://www.migvapor.com/herb-e-micro-vaporizer
7. WASP Vape Pen: https://www.migvapor.com/wasp-wax-vape-pen
8. Volcano Vaporizer: https://www.storzbickel.com/us/en/volcano/
9. Plenty Desktop Vaporizer: https://www.storz-bickel.com/us/en/plenty/
10. Butane cigar torch: https://www.amazon.com/dp/B07CTNM1YC
11. Glass Water Pipe: https://www.amazon.com/dp/B07HF6D8NM

Indoor Grow Equipment and Supplies:

Since the cannabis industry is quickly evolving, keep your eye out on new developments that'll make your indoor grow easier and less costly.

1. iPower Grow Tent: https://www.amazon.com/dp/B00RW2V2HO
2. Woods Manual Timer: https://www.amazon.com/dp/B006LYHDXQ
3. Viparspectra V600: https://www.amazon.com/dp/B019ETLC7M
4. Ledgle Rope Hanger: https://www.amazon.com/dp/B01LWOWBGT
5. Hydrofarm Hot House: https://www.amazon.com/dp/B0006VK68E
6. ViaVolt T5 Grow Light: https://www.amazon.com/dp/B00IPUHEXS
7. Circulating fan: https://www.amazon.com/dp/B000YKC0UY
8. iPower Fan/ Filter Combo: https://www.amazon.com/dp/B00DIGJZ54
9. Humidity/ Temp. Monitor: https://www.amazon.com/dp/B01H1R0K68
10. Taotronics Humidifier: https://www.amazon.com/dp/B01JYIAUEY
11. Compact space heater: https://www.amazon.com/dp/B00I4UVGHO
12. Thermostat controller: https://www.amazon.com/dp/B01MXXBX26

13. Dehumidifier: https://www.amazon.com/dp/B01HXVUT7C
14. Belkin Power Strip: https://www.amazon.com/dp/B000J2EN4S
15. Exhaust Fan Controller: https://www.amazon.com/dp/B0714FFG4F
16. Coco Coir: https://www.amazon.com/dp/B003MOD2HY
17. Smart Pot Containers: https://www.amazon.com/dp/B017WWH7TK
18. MaXX Yield Air Pots: https://www.amazon.com/dp/B017L33NI4
19. Hydrofarm 14" Drip Tray: https://www.amazon.com/dp/B008XOSHR8
20. String Trellis Netting: https://www.amazon.com/dp/B01NBU1VCM
21. Diablo Nutrients: http://diablonutrients.com/products.html
22. Advanced Nutrients: https://www.amazon.com/dp/B0116VEJIA
23. Foxfarm Nutrients: https://www.amazon.com/dp/B000HY2IXQ
24. General Hydroponics: https://www.amazon.com/dp/B017H73708
25. Cal-Mag: https://www.amazon.com/dp/B00F6PJ3M0
26. Bud Candy: https://www.amazon.com/dp/B003OTZ2PW
27. Mycorrhizae: https://www.amazon.com/dp/B00A8PG6RI
28. pH and TDS Meter: https://www.amazon.com/dp/B06XKMH86J
29. pH Calibration Kit: https://www.amazon.com/dp/B017H73794
30. pH Up & Down: https://www.amazon.com/dp/B000BNKWZY
31. Soil Moisture Meter: https://www.amazon.com/dp/B00PTLGKSQ
32. Yellow Sticky Traps: https://www.amazon.com/dp/B01I9KUKLQ
33. SM-90 Growth Fertilizer: https://www.amazon.com/dp/B00CJIZMMC
34. TanLin Pest Control: https://www.amazon.com/dp/B06XNN8VLC
35. Protective Eyewear: https://www.amazon.com/dp/B01MT9NZEQ
36. Pruning Shears: https://www.amazon.com/dp/B00VI2D4Y8
37. Plastic Drinking Cups: https://www.amazon.com/dp/B0792PD6KQ
38. Pocket Microscope: https://www.amazon.com/dp/B00LAX52IQ
39. CoffeeVac canister: https://www.amazon.com/dp/B0046JB136
40. Ona Gel De-Odorizer: https://www.amazon.com/dp/B00AE115UO
41. Precision Pocket Scale: https://www.amazon.com/dp/B01FQRBMZ8
42. CBD / THC Test Kits: http://compassionateanalytics.com
43. Bubble Bags Set: https://www.amazon.com/dp/B00LL6IAWW

26 Finance and Investment Resources to Explore:

Here is a list of the majority of the resources that I've used over the years to help me become a better investor. Some of these are classic guides that have stood the test of time. Should something tickle your fancy, check out those topics that may be of interest.

Secrets of the Millionaire Mind by T. Harv Eker
Publisher: Harper Business (2005)
Hardcover: 224 pages

Power of Focus by Jack Canfield, Mark Victor Hansen and Les Hewitt
Publisher: HCI (2000)
Paperback: 310 pages

The Power Curve by Scott Kyle
Publisher: Nautilus Press (2009)
Hardcover: 256 pages

Trading in the Zone by Mark Douglas
Publisher: Prentice Hall Press (January 1, 2001)
Hardcover: 240 pages

Market Mind Games by Denise Shull
Publisher: McGraw-Hill (2011)
Hardcover: 288 pages

Rich Dad's Guide to Investing by Robert Kiyosaki
Publisher: Time Warner Books (2000)
Paperback: 403 pages

The Millionaire Next Door: The Surprising Secrets of America's Wealthy by
Thomas Stanley & William Danko
Publisher: Taylor Trade Publishing (2010)
Paperback: 272 pages

The Millionaire Maker: Act, Think, and Make Money the Way the Wealthy
Do by Loral Langemeier
Publisher: McGraw-Hill (2005)
Hardcover: 240 pages

Rich Dad's Advisers: Guide to Investing In Gold and Silver: Protect Your
Financial Future by Michael Maloney
Publisher: Business Plus (2008)
Paperback: 240 pages

Getting Back to Even: Your Personal Economic Recovery Plan by James J. Cramer
Publisher: Simon & Schuster (2009)
Hardcover: 352 pages

Options Trading for the Conservative Investor: Increasing Profits without Increasing Risk by Michael C. Thomsett
Publisher: Prentice Hall (2005)
Paperback: 255 pages

Rule #1: The Simple Strategy for Successful Investing in Only 15 Minutes a Week by Phil Town
Publisher: Three Rivers Press (2007)
Paperback: 330 pages

Beating the Street: by Peter Lynch
Publisher: Simon & Schuster (1993)
Hardcover: 318 pages

What Works on Wall Street: The Classic Guide to the Best-Performing Investment Strategies of All Time by James P. O'Shaughnessy
Publisher: McGraw Hill (2012)
Hardcover: 681 pages

Getting Started in Options by Michael Thomsett
Publisher: John Wiley & Sons (2007)
Paperback: 383 pages

Options Made Easy: Your Guide to Profitable Trading by Guy Cohen
Publisher: FT Press (2005)
Hardcover: 335 pages

All About Market Indicators: The Easy Way to Get Started by Michael Sincere Publisher: McGraw Hill (2011)
Paperback: 217 pages

Buy High Sell Higher: Why Buy-AND-Hold Is Dead & Other Investing Lessons from CNBC's "The Liquidator" by Joe Terranova
Publisher: Business Plus (2012)
Hardcover: 261 pages

Buy and Hedge: The 5 Iron Rules for Investing Over the Long Term by Jay Pestrichelli & Wayne Ferbert
Publisher: FT Press (2012)
Hardcover: 289 pages

Exit Strategies for Covered Calls by Alan Ellman
Publisher: Wheatmark (2009)
Paperback: 178 pages

Cashing in on Covered Calls by Alan Ellman
Publisher: SAMR Productions (2007)
Paperback: 392 pages

New Insights on Covered Call Writing by Richard Lehman & Lawrence McMillan
Publisher: Bloomberg Press (2003)
Hardcover: 240 pages

Stock Trader's Almanac by Jeffrey Hirsch & Yale Hirsch
Publisher: John Wiley & Sons
Hardcover: 192 pages

High Probability Trading by Marcel Link
Publisher: McGraw Hill (2003)
Hardcover: 393 pages

Unfair Advantage: The Power of Financial Education by Robert Kiyosaki
Publisher: Plata Publishing (2011)
Paperback: 275 pages

The Millionaire Fastlane by MJ DeMarco
Publisher: Viperion (2011)
Paperback: 322 pages

All the best in your future endeavors!